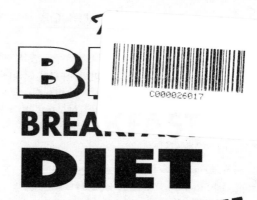

BIG

BREAKFAST

DIET

WARNING!
This book may seriously affect your figure.

ABOUT THE AUTHOR

Eve Cameron is Health and Beauty Director of *Cosmopolitan* magazine and she is the co-author of two other books: *One to One Massage* and *Short Cuts to Looking and Feeling Great*. She eats as she preaches, but admits she could practise a bit more exercise.

Star sign: **Aries with Scorpio rising**
Distinguishing marks: **Tattoo on left hip**
Favourite breakfast: **Porridge**. Beauty tip: **massage left-over porridge over your face to smooth and brighten the complexion**
Lives in: **West London**

The BIG BREAKFAST DIET

Eve Cameron

PAN BOOKS

in association with

Channel Four Television Corporation

and

Planet 24

First published 1994 by
Pan Books
A division of Pan Macmillan Publishers Limited
Cavaye Place London SW10 9PG
and Basingstoke

ISBN 0 330 33514 6

9 8 7 6 5 4 3 2 1

A CIP record for this book is available from the
British Library

Typeset by Parker Typesetting Service, Leicester

Printed and bound in Great Britain by
Cox & Wyman Ltd, Reading, Berkshire

The Big Breakfast television programme is produced for Channel Four
Television by Planet 24 based on an original idea by Charlie Parsons. You can
write to *The Big Breakfast* at 2 Lockkeepers' Cottages, Old Ford Lock,
London E3 2NN.

NOTE: If you have a medical condition or are pregnant, the diet and exercises
described in this book should not be followed without first consulting your
doctor. All guidelines should be read carefully and the author and publisher
cannot accept responsibility for injuries or damage arising out of a failure to
comply with the same.

CONTENTS

AUTHOR'S ACKNOWLEDGEMENTS

The author would like to thank Helen Gummer at Pan Macmillan for her patience and support and for never losing her sense of humour, or at least not letting on that she had; James Strachan at Pan Macmillan for his sense of humour; Fiona Cotter-Craig and Susan Morse at *The Big Breakfast*; Val, Ed, Rob, Ronnie, Jasmine and Lisa from *The Big Breakfast* crew for posing so professionally for the exercise section; Karena and Susan at *Cosmopolitan*; Dorothy and Stephen Purdew, Peter Bissell and the chefs at Henlow Grange Health Farm in Bedfordshire for their expert advice on exercise, plus some great recipes; Paul Connolly, Madeleine Burbidge, Stephen and Jan Mosbacher of Wild Oats and Jane Southern; and last, but definitely not least, my fabulous mum, for all her help and encouragement.

CHAPTER ONE

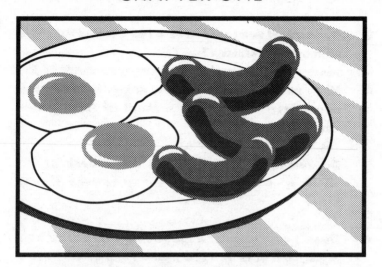

A Breakfast that's Bigger is Better for Your Figure

Are you too big for your boots ... your trousers, your chair, your bed, your *car*? Do our quick quiz and then we'll chew the fat.

1 *Is there a padlock permanently fixed to your fridge door?*

Yes   No

2 *Are you fed up with people asking when the baby's due – and you're not even pregnant?*

Yes   No

3 *Do you feel you could write a book called 101 Ways with Cottage Cheese?*

Yes   No

4 *Have you been on every diet going, including the one where you just eat a sheet of toilet paper every day?*

Yes   No

5 *Do you think you could win the Anorak of the Week spot with all your empty cottage cheese tubs?*

Yes   No

6 *Do you ever wonder if the people who decide how much food goes into pre-packed diet meals have a very sick sense of humour?*

Yes   No

7 *Is your worst nightmare being force-fed cottage cheese?*

Yes   No

8 *Have most diets made you feel light-headed and less than energetic?*

Yes   No

9 *Most diets allow you to snack in between meals . . . on cottage cheese.*

Yes   No

10 *Dieting often seems to cost more than not dieting and you usually end up weighing the same (or more) several months later.*

Yes   No

If you answered yes to any of these, it sounds like you're cottage-cheesed, lettuce-leafed and generally dieted-out. The good news about the Big Breakfast Diet is that:

- ☕ you don't have to eat any cottage cheese – unless you like it
- ☕ it's fun and not boring at all
- ☕ it works

Pull the Other One

Been on diets before? Then you'll probably have noticed that the only pounds you lose are from your pocket. All those 'extras' aren't bye-bye inches, they're special meals or funny foods, videos and 'new improved' books, club memberships, protein drinks and mega-vitamins (because you're virtually starving).

Then there's the absolutely gob-smacking fact that nine times out of ten after you've finished the diet you're fatter, not fitter, than before! This is because many diets are based on being very low-calorie. Your body responds by saying, 'Red alert . . . food shortage' and slows down to conserve energy. The weight you shed is a lot of fluid and a little fat. Stay on a very low-cal diet and you're on the road to ruin as your body then loses lean tissue – and your metabolism drops even lower. Go back to Planet Normal food and your battered old body takes a while to get going again. But, quick as a flash, before you can say Nigel Mansell, all those pounds of flab are making themselves at home again, settling down to watch *Neighbours*.

The Magnificent 7
(Good Reasons to Fight the Flab)

- Big can be beautiful, but if you're really huge, research suggests that you're more likely to have health problems, such as diabetes, strokes, gall bladder disease, high blood pressure and some cancers.
- Being obese can cause problems with your fertility.
- You'll probably live longer if you're not overweight.
- Overload alarm! Eating too much puts extra stress on all your body's systems.
- You won't have to keep letting out your waistbands
- Be slim and you'll be as fast as Keith Chegwin's cameraman.
- Combine diet with exercise, and the natural hormones and chemicals in your body will get working to make you feel ever so HAPPY!

The Big Breakfast *Revolution*

What's different about the *Big Breakfast* diet? Just like *The Big Breakfast* show, the diet is FUN and makes you feel good all day long. It's not a get-slim-quick plan (read: con) though – you'll lose around a healthy 2 pounds a week if you follow the diet exactly. When there's less to lose, you can follow it for a while, use bits of it or adapt it as you wish. It's based on FOUR GOLDEN HOUSE RULES.

Golden House Rule No. 1
ALWAYS EAT UP YOUR BIG BREAKFAST

Yes, it's official, a big breakfast is even better for you than previously thought.

- *Interestingly* . . . eat breakfast and you're less likely to pig out on elevenses.
- *Spookily* . . . not having breakfast may make you more accident-prone.
- *Alarmingly* . . . skip breakfast and you could skip to the bottom of the class. Some studies have shown that kids who always miss out on brekkie have lower academic abilities.
- *Unhealthily* . . . other reports say that non-big-breakfasting kids have higher cholesterol levels — which could be a problem for them in later life.
- *Slimmingly* . . . if you believe that old dieting chestnut that a big breakfast piles on the pounds, chew on this: research in the United States found that when dieters who played hookey at the breakfast table and who weren't losing much weight started having breakfast again, their weight loss started up again too. And, in a French study, it was found that schoolchildren who regularly skipped breakfast were more likely to be overweight than those who had breakfast.
- *Happily* . . . eating a hearty breakfast will help your powers of concentration and make you less likely to be grumpy.
- *Snackingly* . . . if you've filled up on breakfast, you won't be tempted to nibble away all day.

Which all adds up to a lot of sound reasons for Golden House Rule No. 1. And coming up in Chapter 3 there are lots of ideas for all the different things you could be having for breakfast.

Golden House Rule No. 2
BREAKFAST IS BIG, LUNCH IS MEDIUM, DINNER IS SMALL

Remember that old saying 'Breakfast like a king, lunch like a prince and dine like a pauper'? Well, it wasn't invented by someone at *The Big Breakfast*. It makes sense for all the reasons in Golden House Rule No. 1, plus a few others. Your lunch should be healthy and filling to keep you going. Your evening meal should be light and preferably eaten around three hours before going to sleep. The lighter and earlier it is, the more you can burn off and not store as fat. You'll have a better night's sleep, too, if that tum isn't working overtime.

Golden House Rule No. 3
EAT LOTS OF DIFFERENT FOODS, BUT CUT DOWN ON FAT AND SUGAR

You are what you eat. Eat healthily and you'll be more healthy. Eat crap and you'll feel it. Before you start groaning, healthy eating isn't all lettuce and lentils, sandal-wearing and knitting biodegradable yoghurt. It's about:

- eating a wide variety of different foods, especially plenty of fresh vegetables and fruit
- eating less red meat and more lean white meat and fish
- not frying everything that moves

☕ cutting down on sugar and fat

Freeing yourself of fat is particularly important as it can keep your heart healthy, make you feel more energetic and keep you slim. One study has tested a low-fat diet against a calorie-restricted one. After around three months, the women on the low-fat diet had lost twice as much weight as the women on the low-cal one, even though they hadn't been restricting other foods. So the proof is in the pudding – less fat means less 'conventional' dieting.

There's a theory, too, that calories (units of energy) from fat make you fatter than calories from other foods. That's a hard one to explain, but it's along the lines that your body can easily make the fat you eat into the fat you carry around with you, whereas other calories, say from protein, make your body work harder to store them away for a rainy day, so it would rather use them up immediately.

The crunch about eating healthily is that it doesn't just help you to lose weight, it's also a good way to live. The principles in this book are like a trifle:

☕ One layer is that it's a diet that will work for you if followed without any cheating.

☕ The next layer reveals that it's full of healthy eating ideas for the whole family that give sparkling good health, energy and glowing good looks.

☕ Dig into the next layer and you'll find that the principles are an insurance policy for a longer, fitter life.

Golden House Rule No. 4
IF YOU DON'T USE IT, YOU'LL LOSE IT. GET ACTIVE!

Get up off that couch! There's no way you'll ever get in shape without exercise (see Chapter 6).

- If you work out regularly (at least three times a week) you can speed up your metabolism. And you'll burn off more calories.
- Getting moving means getting lean muscle, and lean muscle uses up more calories in the body than flab does.
- Physical activity tones up your physique, giving the flabby bits shape.

A Weighty Question

So do you really need to lose weight? Some people call themselves fat when they aren't really – their clothes are just a bit tight and they think they could lose a couple of pounds. Then there's overweight. That's when you can't see your toes any more, everything's dropping by an inch a year and you need a completely new wardrobe. And then there's obese. Obesity means the only clothes you can fit into are kaftans and your health could be in danger. Remember the Fat Man in *Monty Python's The Meaning of Life*? After eating too much, he had one last wafer-thin mint. Then he exploded. Don't let this happen to you.

Here are two ways to work out roughly what weight is right for you:

THE BODY MASS INDEX

Unless you're brilliant at sums, doing this bit of arithmetic will probably burn off quite a few calories by itself.

$$\frac{\text{weight in kilograms}}{\text{height in metres} \times \text{height in metres}} = \text{BMI}$$

Well done if your BMI is between 18.1 and 23.6 if you're a woman and between 20.1 and 25 if you're a man. More than 25, you're overweight. More than 30, technically you're obese.

CHECK-YOUR-WEIGHT CHARTS

(see pages 10 and 11)

Keep it in the Family

Is it true that people get fat because they eat too much and don't get enough exercise? Very often, yes, though sometimes hormone treatment, the Pill and food allergies can also make you balloon. Your genes play a part too, but remember things like over-eating can run in families.

Chart 1. Guidelines in metric for body weight (Bray, 1979: based on Metropolitan Life Insurance tables, 1960). The minimum level for diagnosing obesity is taken as 20 per cent above the upper limit of the acceptable weight range.

Height without shoes (m)	Men Weight without clothes (kg)			Women Weight without clothes (kg)		
	Acceptable average	Acceptable weight range	Obese	Acceptable average	Acceptable weight range	Obese
1.45				46.0	42–53	64
1.48				46.5	42–54	65
1.50				47.0	43–55	66
1.52				48.5	44–57	68
1.54				49.5	44–58	70
1.56				50.4	45–58	70
1.58	55.8	51–64	77	51.3	46–59	71
1.60	57.6	52–65	78	52.6	48–61	73
1.62	58.6	53–66	79	54.0	49–62	74
1.64	59.6	54–67	80	55.4	50–64	77
1.66	60.6	55–69	83	56.8	51–65	77
1.68	61.7	56–71	85	58.1	52–66	78
1.70	63.5	58–73	88	60.0	53–67	79
1.72	65.0	59–74	89	61.3	55–69	80
1.74	66.5	60–75	90	62.6	56–70	83
1.76	68.0	62–77	92	64.0	58–72	84
1.78	69.4	64–79	95	65.3	59–74	86
1.80	71.0	65–80	96			89
1.82	72.6	66–82	98			
1.84	74.2	67–84	101			
1.86	75.8	69–86	103			
1.88	77.6	71–88	106			
1.90	79.3	73–90	108			
1.92	81.0	75–93	112			
BMI	22.0	20.1–25.0	30.0	20.8	18.1–23.8	29.0

Chart 2. Guidelines in non-metric for body weight (Bray, 1979: based on Metropolitan Life Insurance tables, 1960). The minimum level for diagnosing obesity is taken as 20 per cent above the upper limit of the acceptable weight range.

Height without shoes (ft, in)	Men			Women		
	Acceptable average	Acceptable weight range	Obese	Acceptable average	Acceptable weight range	Obese
4 10				102	92–119	143
4 11				104	94–122	146
5 0				107	96–125	150
5 1				110	99–128	154
5 2	123	112–141	169	113	102–131	157
5 3	127	115–144	173	116	105–134	161
5 4	130	118–148	178	120	108–138	166
5 5	133	121–152	182	123	111–142	170
5 6	136	124–156	187	128	114–146	175
5 7	140	128–161	193	132	118–150	180
5 8	145	132–166	199	136	122–154	185
5 9	149	136–170	204	140	126–158	190
5 10	153	140–174	209	144	130–163	196
5 11	158	144–179	215	148	134–168	202
6 0	162	148–184	221	152	138–173	208
6 1	166	152–189	227			
6 2	171	156–194	233			
6 3	176	160–199	239			
6 4	181	164–204	245			

(Source: The Royal College of Physicians: *Obesity*)

The Flip Side – Going Too Far

Just as being larger than life is bad for your health, so is being a skinny weakling. And it's really stupid to get that way through anorexia or bulimia. Being incredibly thin doesn't mean that (a) people will like you more, (b) you'll fall in love and live happily ever after, or (c) that you'll get that dream job. What having an eating disorder means is that you have emotional problems which will end up as a very serious physical condition. Whoever or whatever you blame – your parents, diet books, advertising, skinny models – please get help. Talk to a doctor, a friend, a relative or a teacher NOW. You won't have the stamina to keep up with *The Big Breakfast* if you don't look after Number One.

Giving Up is Hard to Do . . .

Chocolate fudge cake, says Tom O' Connor.
Ice cream and chocolates, sighs Bella Emberg.
Chocolate, confesses Toyah Wilcox.
Indian food, particularly chicken tikka masala in that shockingly red, unnatural sauce, reports Jonathon Ross.
Crisps, admits Pat Cash.

CELEBRITY DIETING DISASTERS AND TIPS

Pat Cash

Boo: 'Just after I got married, my wife Emily was cooking big roasts every two or three days. This is the only time I have been overweight.'

Hooray: 'Eat pasta – lots of it. And no butter, or only a little of it, on bread and other food.'

Toyah Wilcox

Boo: 'A boiled eggs diet – I didn't go to the loo for the next seven days.'

Hooray: 'Eat what you want, when you want, never weigh yourself and don't look in the mirror.'

Bella Emberg

Boo: 'When I was twenty-six I made myself ill trying to slim.'

Hooray: 'Say no to sweet things.'

Back in the (OLD) USSR –

There's an old Russian saying that goes something like this:

Breakfast you eat for yourself
Lunch you share with a friend
Dinner you give to your enemy

DID YOU KNOW?

In Japan, many adults eat breakfast and lunch but skip dinner, having a cup or two of sake instead.

Just for the Record

Coming up in the breakfast, lunch and dinner sections you'll find plenty of tasty, healthy, waistline-conscious recipes which we hope you'll use and enjoy. But this book is also a veritable little gold mine of healthy cooking and eating ideas, guidelines and tips – the aim being that you can put all this knowledge into practice with your own recipes, making new and improved versions.

CHAPTER TWO

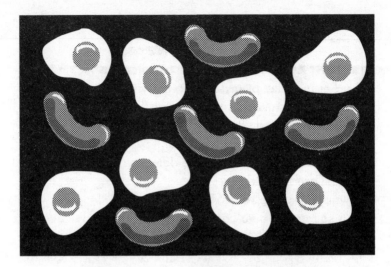

Super-Hints on Home Economics

(Your indispensable guide to looking and feeling disgustingly healthy, plus having snake-like hips, and skin, teeth and hair that look fabulous)

Here's an A–Z crash-course in nutritional know-how. As well as some basic dietary guidelines which you should know, there are also some handy hints and surprising facts in this section. So don't skip it.

A is for . . .

STRAIGHT ACE Deal yourself the best hand by making sure your diet includes plenty of the vital vitamins A, C and E. More and more research is suggesting that they:

- 🍵 protect against cancers
- 🍵 lower the risk of heart disease
- 🍵 protect against age-related damage, such as cataracts and arthritis
- 🍵 may even help your skin look younger for longer

Good sources of beta-carotene (which your body converts into vitamin A) include spinach, broccoli, apricots, carrots and tomatoes. For vitamin C, go for baked potatoes, oranges, grapefruits, blackcurrants, Brussels sprouts and parsley (parsley sauce has never been so thrilling, as Angus Deayton might say). Best bets for vitamin E include sunflower oil, wheatgerm, almonds, egg yolk and peanut butter.

AN APPLE A DAY, so they say, keeps the doctor away (like vampires and garlic?). Anyway, apples are good to snack on when you're dieting. They're fibre-rich, so they fill you up faster, for longer and more virtuously than a couple of biscuits.

ALCOHOL Big boozers are losers in the slimming stakes. Alcohol helps pile on the pounds, and if you drink too much you'll end up with a fat red nose too, not to mention a possible whole host of other rather more serious problems. Experts are always arguing about exactly how much is good/bad for you. At present the safe recommended guidelines per week are 21 units or under for men and 14 units or under for women. A unit is half a regular strength lager/beer, one glass of wine or a single spirit measure. Healthwise, moderation is, of course, the key. Dietwise, cut *down* if you can't cut out.

B is for . . .

A SENSE OF BALANCE A balanced diet means eating a variety of different foods. On a daily basis, get the balance right by mixing the food groups. For example, don't eat meat for breakfast, lunch and dinner, or have three egg-based meals. Not only does eating plenty of different things give you maximum points nutritionally, it also beats the boredom factor.

B COMPLEX No, this won't make your character more interesting, nor will it turn your nose a millimetre to the right, explode your boss's dishwasher during an important dinner party or even get you on *The Big Breakfast*. However, the B-complex vitamins do work together to help your body do things such as release energy from food and assist the functions of the nervous system. These vitamins are found in, for example, wholegrain foods, fish, pulses, yeast extracts (e.g. Marmite) and offal.

MORE BISCUITS WITH YOUR TEA, VICAR? Pigging out on biscuits sends you to the bottom of the class. Full of sugar and fat, they do nothing for you nutritionally and nor will they help you lose weight. Don't buy them, so they're not there begging to be eaten.

BUTTER WOULDN'T MELT IN HER MOUTH Butter isn't banned from this diet, as it is in many others. But there is a little bit of compromising to be done. Butter is OK on your breakfast toast (there's nothing more boring or depressing than dry toast, is there?) or in the occasional sandwich in the evening if you don't go for low-fat spread. However, butter is fattening, so it's banned from cooking. And equally, there's no cheating with putting great lumps of it on your vegetables or in baked potatoes. Incidentally, did you know that margarine is no less fattening than butter? Low-fat spreads are the ones with fewer calories.

C is for . . .

CABBAGE PATCH Everyone's fave at school (*not!*) comes highly recommended by the Japanese. As well as making you a better karaoke artiste, they reckon it could also lower your risk of colon cancer by as much as 66 per cent. Mmmm, make mine a double helping . . .

MUCH ADO ABOUT CALORIES Calories are the units that measure the amount of energy you get from foods. They are mentioned in this book, but never to do with calorie-counting or calorie-controlling.

CHOLESTEROL CORRECTNESS We're just mentioning this because cholesterol is a word that's bandied about a lot. It's quite hard to spell: close your eyes and see if you can. In one way it's good for you, helping your body do important things like hormone-building, fat-digesting and vitamin-D-making. But it's bad news when you have too much of a particular kind of it, which is the stuff that gets stuck in your arteries and increases your risk of a heart attack. Saturated fat (in lard, red meat, cakes, etc – *see* Fats and Figures, page 20) raises the 'bad cholesterol' – another good reason not to eat too much of it. Try to make it less than 10 per cent of your daily diet. Watch out for 'hydrogenated vegetable fat' too. You might think it sounds healthy, but it's actually high in saturates.

And, just for the record, high cholesterol is not the only risk factor for a heart attack. Add being overweight, smoking and heavy boozing.

IT AIN'T WHAT YOU COOK IT'S THE WAY THAT YOU COOK IT Say yes to things like:

- *steaming* – especially good for root veggies, broccoli and cauliflower, for getting the most flavour and nutrients. You can get special steaming saucepans or a steaming basket that sits on the pan. Check the water is boiling before you get the veggies all hot and steamy.
- *stir-frying* – back in China they know wok's wok. Stir-frying cooks vegetables fast in very little oil, so they lose few of their nutrients. Great for tasty fish, seafood and meat too.
- *pressure-cooking* – this cooks vegetables at a high temperature very quickly in very little water, therefore keeping them power-packed.

Remember, overcooked vegetables are 'orrible. Boil them to death and it's no wonder no one wants to eat them.

D is for . . .

DISCIPLINE, DOWN YOUR DOORSTEP, which you're going to need if you're serious about losing weight. Yes, it would be nice if you could get slim sitting on the sofa eating Mars bars, but life ain't like that. To lose weight you really have to want to do it and be prepared to work at it, through changing your eating habits and getting some kind of exercise every day.

E is for . . .

EATING OUT doesn't have to be the death of your diet, if it's an occasional treat. There are two possible approaches. Either have exactly what you want and enjoy it, but promise yourself that you won't feel guilty or depressed in the morning (and that you'll get straight back to your good habits). Or be very mature and make some thought-through choices. For example, say no to frying and choose instead from the baked, broiled/grilled or steamed dishes. If they come with buttery or creamy sauces, have none or just a spoonful. At the Chinese or Indian ask for plain boiled rice and go for chicken, fish or seafood cooked in the simplest, driest way, like chicken tikka. Again, watch the sauces, they are potentially very fattening. Beware coconutty ones in particular – they'll be sitting on your hips almost as fast as they pass your lips. So does that mean hasta la vista piña coladas too? $2 + 2 = 4$.

F is for . . .

FATS AND FIGURES Eating a diet high in fats is one road to obesity. Along the way you also increase the risk of health problems such as heart disease. Britain has one of the highest rates of heart disease in the world, which is largely (though not totally) due to our massive intake of saturated fat.

Fats do have some uses, though: for instance, as an energy source and player in many other bodily functions. Basically we just eat too much of the wrong sort. And the sad fact for dieters is that all too often the fat you eat turns into the fat you wear. The fats to cut down on in particular are saturated fats – ones from animal sources. Unsaturated fats come from vegetable sources (like sunflower and olive oils) and from oily fish, such as mackerel, salmon, trout and herrings. These fats are the good guys, because they can actually help protect against heart disease. Current guidelines suggest not more than 30% of our diet is made up of fats (10% saturated and 20% unsaturated).

EAT MORE FIBRE AND YOU TOO CAN BE FLUSHED WITH SUCCESS The fibre in foods like beans, fruit, salads, vegetables and cereals cleans out your pipes, helping to push out waste products. Regular flushings help beat bowel problems and things you wouldn't like to own up to, like piles. The bulk in fibre tends to make you feel fuller too, which is why fibre-rich foods are a double-whammy for dieters.

A word of warning: too much fibre too soon and you'll probably end up full of gas with an attractively bloated tummy to boot. Up your fibre intake gradually.

FARTING Beans always cause a snigger because of their association with wind. Sometimes they give you a cold after your duvet has floated 3 inches above your body all night. If you cook them properly, though (check how to on the packet), they're less likely to make you blow off. Most importantly, beans, together with peas and lentils, are a good source of fibre, protein, iron and other nutrients. They're a good, cheap alternative to meat and fish too.

OUT OF THE FRYING PAN INTO THE BIN? As well as cooking in healthier ways, such as grilling, check the state of your frying pan. If your old pan is so worn that you need to use double fat to keep things from sticking, now's the time to part with it. As a commitment to the *Big Breakfast* diet, buy yourself a brand-spanking-new *non-stick* pan. The non-stick bit is important — it means that when you do occasionally use your frying pan, you'll be able to cook with little or no fat.

G is for . . .

EAT YOUR GREENS Yes, that phrase has come back from childhood to haunt you together with (if you're not eating them) 'You're old enough to know better . . .'

H is for . . .

HUNGER Sometimes we think we're hungry when actually we're thirsty. If in between meals you start to feel bored and peckish, down a couple of glasses of water. You may find it's all you need.

I is for . . .

IMAGINE (at frequent intervals) how much fitter and lither you're going to be . . .

J is for . . .

JUNK FOOD An occasional junk food meal will do you no harm at all. The danger is when it's a regular fat-filled feature of your diet.

K is for . . .

KITCHEN Make yours a diet-friendly zone. Check the Swap

Shop list below, incorporate the rest of the A–Z knowledge and spring clean your cupboards and fridge. Keep stocked up on the good and healthy choices and don't replace those diet-defeating extras.

L is for . . .

LIQUID REFRESHMENT Drinking plenty of fluids is essential, whether you're dieting or not. Best of all is water (*see* Water Really Works) followed by sugar-free fruit and vegetable juices and herbal teas. Fizzy drinks contain a lot of sugar – some colas, for example, have as much as a teeth-rotting seven teaspoons. If you like your drinks fizzy, go for diet versions or, better still, just mix fizzy water with natural fruit juice. Watch out for fruit 'drinks' and squashes as they've usually got added sugar too. Tea and coffee are only slimline when they're black or made with skimmed milk and when sugar-free. If you're a sugar fiend, try a sugar substitute. Five cuppas a day is probably enough. Tea can actually bung you up in the toilet department, so it's best not to drink too much.

M is for . . .

MEAT is a good source of iron and other minerals, protein and some B vitamins, but bear in mind that red meat is also high in saturated fat, as are meat pies and sausages (shame), so they're best avoided by slimmers. There is room for meat in your diet, but try not to have it every day. Even then, choose lean meat and trim off all visible fat, making it look like your favourite Chippendale. White meat, like chicken and turkey, is already lower in fat, but you should always take the skin off so that it's less fattening. (Throwing away the remaining meat also helps cut down on fat – that's a joke, birdbrain!) Cut down on the quantity you serve up too. Instead of the meat being the main focus of your plate, accompanied by a few vegetables and potatoes, swap things around so the meat is a small, tasty accompaniment to your vegetables or salad, potatoes, noodles, rice or whatever.

N is for . . .

HOLD YOUR NOSE! In recent studies in Holland, psychologists found that simply smelling cakes and confectionery was enough to drive dieters to despair.

O is for . . .

ONE LUMP OR TWO? Sugar is a bit like the daily papers if you're famous – one minute they build you up, the next they knock you down. A bit of sugar temporarily lifts you, then messes with your blood sugar levels to make them fall lower than they were before you had the sugar-fix. The result: feeling hungry, grouchy and tired.

Sugar is also a selfish partner because it gives you lots of calories without any nutrients to write home about. If you want to lose weight, cut sugar out. If you can't make a clean break, do it gradually. Having said that, don't get a one-track mind. You really don't have to face the rest of your life without ever having another cream éclair.

P is for . . .

PORKY PIES Despite what's on the bestseller lists, don't be fooled by Big Fat Dieting Lies. Classics include:
- grapefruit with every meal helping to burn up calories
- low-carbohydrate, high-protein diets – you'll lose a lot of fluid, but then . . . (*see* Up and Down Like a Yo-Yo).
- spot reduction – this has probably got more to do with acne control than losing weight from specific areas. While the experts do argue about this one, as a general rule you lose from the tummy first, then the face, then the upper back and then the hips and thighs.

GET PUMPIN' WITH PUMPKIN SEEDS According to one nutrition expert, a handful of pumpkin seeds each day could up your sexual performance, increase a woman's fertility and help save men from prostate surgery.

Q is for . . .

QUIDS IN Following the *Big Breakfast* healthier diet won't mean having to take out a mortgage.

R is for . . .

RELAX Romford wasn't built in a day. You will be slimmer, trimmer and healthier, but it takes time. With the *Big Breakfast* diet you'll have lasting results. Don't fall for the crash-diet cowboys: they might promise to make your day, but they're all mouth and no trousers. We've said it before and we'll say it again – the only way to lose weight, stay in shape and feel fab is to diet the healthy *Big Breakfast* way.

S is for . . .

HAVE SAFE SNACKS If you feel peckish between meals, have a little something – no, not a beef, pork and pepperoni with five different kinds of cheese pizza. Cakes and biscuits, lumps of cheese and the like are out too. Safe snacks include fruit, raw vegetables, say with a bit of plain yoghurt dip, 'diet' yoghurts with lower fat and artificial sweeteners and crispbreads with low-fat spreads . . .

STRESS BELLY Did you know that, according to one piece of research, if you can't deal with stress you could be more likely to get a fat tummy? So, if you're a big-bellied stress mess, try yoga. Fascinatingly, other research has shown that women who smoke are also more likely to develop tubby tummies. So, if you're a female, smoking stress mess with a doubly tubby tummy, try yoga and quit smoking.

SWAP SHOP This is all about making healthy, mature, figure-happy choices when you're at the supermarket. Choices like:

- canned fruit in syrup *swap for* canned fruit in natural juice with no added sugar
- canned fish in oil *swap for* canned fish in brine or water
- marmalade and jams *swap for* sugar-free or reduced-sugar jams
- lard and other cooking oils *swap for* sunflower or olive oil
- mayonnaise, salad cream and other dressings *swap for* the lower fat or 'lite' versions
- cream *swap for* low-fat crème fraîche or fromage frais

- regular flavoured yoghurts *swap for*   low-fat, low-sugar 'diet' versions
- whole milk *swap for*   skimmed milk
- cakes and biscuits   *swap for*   trimmer thighs

T is for . . .

I CAN RESIST ANYTHING EXCEPT TEMPTATION So wrote the wit Oscar Wilde who knew that if he had a packet of chocolate Hobnobs in the house, he'd eat them. The moral = if you don't buy all those dieting no-nos, they won't be there to tempt you in moments of weakness.

U is for . . .

IT'S UNIVERSAL AND UNISEX The *Big B* diet is politically correct and works for both men and women and those who are vertically, folicley, aesthetically – and all the other -lys you can think of – challenged. It's also not downwardly ageist – whilst kids shouldn't go on a weight loss diet, unless recommended to by a doctor, the healthy eating principles of the *BB* diet, such as eating less fat, can apply to them too.

V is for . . .

VAIT FOR IT, VINEGAR Did you know that drinking vats of vinegar was one of the cures for obesity in the 1500s? But don't try this one at home. Rather than being fat-busting, it could be fatal!

VEGETARIANS tend to have lower blood cholesterol levels and a higher fibre intake than meat-eaters. However, iron can sometimes be a problem, though vegetarians usually eat plenty of fruit and veg containing vitamin C which helps its absorption. B12, one of the B complex (*see* page 17), can also be a bit low in vegetarians, so a supplement may be a good idea. A healthy, clever combination on a vegetarian plate could include beans and pulses with wholegrains — yes, beans on toast are brilliant — and things like cereals with milk and vegetables and potatoes with cheese sauce. All lower-fat types of dairy products, naturally. You wouldn't want to end up a porky herbivore, would you?

W is for . . .

WHOLEMEAL BREAD AND BROWN RICE OK, you may well laugh (cringe?) and think they're only for sandal-wearing veggie hippies, but you should try them, if not for the health benefits, then because they actually taste a whole-meal lot better than the refined white stuff. Besides, aren't you forgetting your large collection of Jim Morrison memorabilia? And the fact that you too used to wear orange flares with a paisley belt? If you have to have white bread, buy reasonable quality, enhanced with seeds on top. Granary, while not as health-boosting as wholemeal, is a good half-way house. Brown rice is yummy, with loads more flavour than white. Try wholemeal pasta too — it's really groovy, man.

WATER REALLY WORKS We need water to stay alive, for one thing. Most of us should drink more to flush out our systems, and some experts say we can boost our energy levels, too, if we drink eight glasses a day. Others say it helps clear spotty skin. It won't hurt anyway. Tea and coffee don't count as water, though, because they are 'diuretics' and actually flush water out of the body so it can't do its thing. You don't have to cut out tea and coffee, just drink plain water in addition.

X is for . . .

X-CELLENT Just a few more letters to digest.

Y is for . . .

UP AND DOWN LIKE A YO-YO This is all too often the story with dieting. One theory goes that when you go on a serious calorie-restricted diet your body goes into starvation mode, slowing down its metabolism to conserve energy. As well as making you light-headed and less than energetic, this kind of dieting makes your body want to hold on to fat supplies. You lose a little weight, but it will be mostly fluid at first. Then, start eating normally and your slowed metabolism takes a while to get going again, resulting in weight gain. And so the pattern goes on.

Z is for . . .

THINK ZINC . . . come again? Did you know that if a man has sex a lot, he could be low on zinc? Apparently each ejaculation contains something like 5 milligrams (the daily recommended intake is 15 milligrams). Do it three times a day on a regular basis and he could well end up short on zinc (as well as pretty knackered). Zinc is naturally found in fish, meat, poultry, seafood, wholegrain foods, egg yolk and seeds and is important for maintaining bones, muscles and hormone levels.

ZAG'S FAVOURITE COLOUR IS PURPLE This might not help your diet, but it could help you to make friends and influence people, not least because you'd have something else to talk about apart from your diet.

CHAPTER THREE

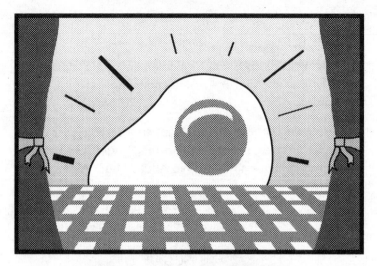

Rise and Dine

Always eat breakfast and make it BIG. You know what will happen if you skip it – you'll be all sleepy, accident-prone, and probably fatter as well because you won't be able to resist an elevenses of a packet of Jaffa Cakes.

In this chapter there are lots of suggestions for what you might like to eat for breakfast. You may have your own ideas too, which is fine – self-expression is encouraged! But do please stick to the healthy principles in this book. Fat and sugar can be a particular temptation at 7.30 a.m. – think of sausage sandwiches, croissants and Danish pastries . . . now forget all about them.

Here's an at-a-glance guide to swapping the breakfasts you might be eating for the breakfasts you *should* be eating:

Instead of	***Go for***
Toasted white bread, with lots of butter and jam or marmalade	Wholemeal bread with just a little butter or low-fat spread, plus sugar-free jam
Sugar-coated cereals or cereals with several extra spoonfuls of sugar and full-fat milk	Sugar-free cereals, such as Shredded Wheat, Grape Nuts, No Added Sugar Alpen, Jordan's Special Recipe Muesli, or make your own muesli. Have them with skimmed milk or yoghurt and NO EXTRA SUGAR
Fried eggs	Boiled eggs
Porridge with cream or full-fat milk and sugar	Porridge made with skimmed milk or water, or a combination of the two. Use sugar-free jam to sweeten or a sugar substitute
Shop-bought cakes and pastries	Our 'Go Bananas' Bread (page 40)
The fully fried full works traditional breakfast	Our less fattening Cholesterol Get Losterol Breakfast (page 44) – occasionally
Nothing	A Big Breakfast

And now for some special *Big Breakfast* recipes for the most important meal of the day.

The Big Chill Breakfast

No wonder the three bears were cross when they found someone had been at their steaming bowls of porridge. They knew that getting your oats on a regular basis gives extra vitality, ups your fibre intake and fills you up without making you fat. As well as being cheap and cheerful, porridge is especially good in the winter when it feels as though the next ice age has arrived and you can actually warm your hands at the fridge door. It'll make you glow inside and out.

- Use 50 g/2 oz or 6 tablespoons of oats per person. A non-dieting Big Lad can have an ounce or two more.

- Traditionally, porridge is cooked with water – this is, of course, best for slimmers too. But, if wet and watery traditions aren't your style, go instead for skimmed milk or a mixture of skimmed milk and water. No excuses for using whole milk – that's for the under fives only.

- *Sweet nothings.* If you have to add some sweetness to your porridge, try a spoonful of sugar-free or reduced-sugar jam, available in most supermarkets.

- *Pass the salt, or pass it up?* Pinch the habit from the Scots if you like a wee bit of salt with your oats. Otherwise, use your salt in the bathroom as a body scrub. Just dampen it slightly and massage over dry skin, from your ankles to your neck. Shower or bathe off.

- *Added value.* Build up interest with a handful of raisins, chopped dried fruit, a banana or a few nuts and seeds thrown into your porridge.

Here's a **PORRIDGE SUPER-HINT** from Tom O'Connor: 'When I have the grandchildren over, they have a dabble of about two or three different cereals. I take the leftovers and chuck them in a bowl of porridge.' Er, thanks, Tom, that sounds lovely. Next time, why not let the grandchildren do the cooking?

DID YOU KNOW?

Oats can sometimes help eczema. As well as just chucking a handful in the bath (which gets very messy), you can also tie up some oats in a muslin bag and hang them under the tap while the water's running. They help to calm the itchy, inflamed skin.

The 'Behind Enemy Lines' Breakfast

Cellulite – the dimply, lumpy, fatty bits that are a woman's thighs' worst enemy – is hard to fight. Strategies include exercise, massage, drinking lots of water and following a simple low-fat and additive-free diet. This breakfast gets you behind enemy lines, working from the inside, with the sort of things that should help not hinder the battle.

🍴 *A Scouting Party:* lead the way with a cup of hot water with freshly squeezed lemon juice. Many experts believe this cleanses and detoxifies the system.

🍴 *Mission Possible:* get together a crack-team of fresh fruits (as much as you want) and chop them up into a fruit salad. Add 2–3 tablespoons plain yoghurt – look out for the codewords 'live' or 'bio', indicating that these yoghurts have beneficial bacteria for great gut reactions.

ιοι *Double Agent:* many experts suggest saying 'niet' to coffee and tea (and alcohol too) when you're trying to combat cellulite, and defecting instead to herbal teas.

Boo: Men don't get cellulite.

Hooray: Even skinny women can get cellulite.

Doctors in the UK think cellulite is all a figment of women's imaginations. *Nuls points.* In France, however, doctors accept that it exists. Jolly good show.

BRUSH UP YOUR SKIN

Here's a cheap trick for nuking that orange-peel skin. Get a natural bristle brush and, for a few minutes every morning, sweep it (dry) over your body from your feet to your neck. Use long, firm strokes and always work towards your heart.

The Lovers' Breakfast

Sensual smoked salmon, caressing caviar and cream cheese on a bed of beautiful blinis ... This one's for special occasions, to share with someone gorgeous. Best eaten in bed.

Blinis

Russian in origin, real blinis are made with buckwheat flour
and yeast. They're smaller and thicker than our pancakes,
looking more like American ones. Vlad and Olga traditionally eat their blinis with sour cream and caviar. Plus, of
course, a shot of vodka.

For 6–8 blinis

50 g/2 oz 81 per cent plain brown or wholemeal flour
*50 g/2 oz buckwheat flour (if you can't find it go for
    either of the above. But, if you do this, you'll need
    more water. You may have to add an extra 25 ml/
    1 fl. oz)*
*1 level teaspoon easy-blend yeast (available in
    supermarkets)*
100 ml/4 fl. oz warm water
1 egg, separated
butter
a pinch of salt

1 Mix the flours, salt and yeast. Add the water gradually
until you have a creamy, thickish consistency.

2 Cover and leave to rise for about 40 minutes, or until it
roughly doubles in bulk. This gives you a good oppor-
tunity to have a cuddle, a massage or read the paper.
Or, put it in a bowl, cover and leave in the fridge
overnight. If you do this, you'll have to take the mixture
out again first thing in the morning to allow it to return
to room temperature and rise a little, say for about half
an hour.

3   Beat the yolk of the egg into the mixture.

4   Whisk up the egg white until it's at its peak, then fold it into the mixture. Leave again for about 20 minutes. You could now catch up on those things you didn't do while the blini mixture was rising.

5   To make the blinis, heat a little bit of butter in a large non-stick frying pan. Drop a tablespoon of the mixture into the pan, which should be on a medium heat. As the mixture doesn't spread much, you should be able to do 2 or 3 at once. Cook them for 2–3 minutes on each side.

6   Keep the finished blinis warm in a preheated oven at its lowest setting while you cook the rest.

7   Serve each blini with a couple of slices of smoked salmon and a dollop of low-fat or 'light' cream cheese or plain fromage frais. For extra oomph, put a sprinkling of dill on the salmon and a spoonful of caviar on the cream cheese.

Blinis are brilliant because
>   you can eat them with anything you like, really, savoury or sweet
>   and
>   they freeze well and can be warmed up

FAMOUS FIVE APHRODISIACS – *True or False?*

Oysters √	Figs √	Fish Fingers ×
Spinach ×	Custard creams ×	

The White-On Breakfast

Yoghurt has an international flavour. The Russians, for instance, drink it as 'kiefer', while the Indians mix it with cucumber in 'raita'. And, if you buy the pots marked 'live' or 'active', it has a culture all of its own. Easily digestible (unlike some of the jokes in this book), it's good for the tummy as it contains beneficial bacteria. It's got protein and calcium too. Here's how to transform plain yoghurt into something stunning.

For 1 person, use 1 regular-sized pot of natural yoghurt and add 4 of the following:

☞ *50 g/2 oz wheatberries (also called wholegrain wheat), soaked and cooked (see page 42)*
☞ *50 g/2 oz rolled oats*
☞ *25 g/1 oz wheatgerm*
☞ *50 g/2 oz bran*
☞ *3 tablespoons regular breakfast cereal*
☞ *1 tablespoon pine kernels, sunflower seeds or pumpkin seeds*
☞ *1 tablespoon slivered almonds*
☞ *25 g/1 oz sultanas or raisins*
☞ *1 piece of fresh fruit, in season*
☞ *1 small tin of peaches, pears or pineapple (in natural juice with no added sugar)*
☞ *1 stewed or puréed apple with a sprinkle of cinnamon*
☞ *50 g/2 oz chopped dried fruit*
☞ *if you need extra sweetness, try a spoonful of sugar-free fruit jam*

FEED YOUR FACE... WITH YOGHURT

For a messy, but fun and skin-smoothing face mask, try this:

For dry skin, mix two tablespoonfuls of yoghurt with the yolk of an egg. For oily skin, mix the yoghurt with a few drops of lemon juice. First put a hot (not boiling) damp flannel on your face for a few minutes. Then apply the yoghurt mix and leave for 15 minutes or so. Try not to move or it will go everywhere! Rinse off with warm water.

SUPERDRINK

To get the most from your meal, have a glass of orange juice with it – it helps with iron absorption.

A Caribbean Breakfast

There'll be no lumps in the way of your limbo-dancing after this typically tropical breakfast – a calypso-singing, ripe and juicy exotic fruit salad, plus an apple and banana bread that you don't have to go all the way to Barbados for. This combination is guaranteed to give you a sunny outlook.

For the fruit salad, simply mix up as much as you fancy of tropical fruits such as papaya, pineapple, mango, banana, starfruit, oranges and lychees.

'Go Bananas' Apple and Banana Bread

1 apple, peeled and sliced
450 g/1 lb wholemeal flour
15 g/½ oz fresh yeast, or if you can't get fresh use
    1 sachet of easy-blend yeast and follow the
    instructions for mixing on the packet
150 ml/¼ pint warm water
50 g/2 oz sugar (or equivalent sugar substitute)
1 tablespoon ground cinnamon
½ tablespoon ground nutmeg
a pinch of salt
50 g/2 oz raisins or sultanas
2 medium-sized bananas, mashed
rind of 1 lemon, grated

1 Cook the apple in a saucepan with a drop of water on a low heat until soft. Then purée and leave to cool.

2 Mix 120 g/4 oz of the flour with the fresh yeast and warm water and put it somewhere warm until it gets frothy. (If using easy-blend yeast, put it in a bowl with all the flour, sugar, spices, salt and raisins or sultanas. Then add the water and stir.)

3 Put the rest of the flour, the sugar, spices and all things nice, the salt and raisins or sultanas in a bowl.

4 Stir the yeast mixture into the bowl, together with the apple purée, banana and lemon rind. Beat and blend.

5 Now put the mixture into 2 greased loaf tins. When the mixture has risen to the tops of the tins bake in the oven for around 35 minutes on 190°C/375°F/Gas Mark 5.

Top Banana Quiz

Questions

1. Name the girl trio who had a bunch of hits including 'Venus' and 'Really Saying Something'.

2. Whose theme tune started, 'One banana, two banana, three banana, four'?

3. What sounds a bit like banana, but you don't eat it, you wear it round your head?

4. How many bananas are there in the average bunch?

5. In Australian slang what do you call someone who comes from Queensland?

6. What is the name of the banana-loving King of the Swingers in *The Jungle Book*?

Answers

1 Bananarama 2 The Banana Splits 3 Bandana 4 Pass 5 A bananalander 6 Louis

Mega-Mix Muesli

Surprisingly, that healthy favourite, muesli, comes from the land that's just cuckoo about chocolate. Invented by a Swiss doctor to help his patients eat their way back to health, muesli now comes in lots of different mixes. If buying it pre-packed, check it has no added sugar for your flab to yodel about. Here's a recipe for making your own.

Serves 2

50 g/2 oz wheatberries (also called wholegrain wheat)
  or substitute 25 g/1 oz wheatgerm
50 g/2 oz rolled oats
1 tablespoon sultanas or raisins
1 tablespoon seeds, such as pumpkin or sunflower
1 tablespoon chopped almonds
25 g/1 oz ready-to-eat dried apricots
2 small eating apples, peeled and grated
3 tablespoons skimmed milk or plain yoghurt

1 If using wheatberries, which are chewy and yummy, you will need to soak and cook them first. Soak overnight in a bowl of water, then put in a pan with fresh water. Bring to the boil, then simmer for around 50 minutes or until soft.

2 You could soak the oats with the sultanas or raisins overnight too – just put them in a bowl with a couple of tablespoons of water or orange or apple juice. If you don't want to do this, simply put the oats, sultanas or raisins, seeds, almonds and apricots in a bowl with 2 tablespoonfuls of water or juice.

3 Add the wheatberries and grated apple to the oats mixture.

4 Top up with the skimmed milk or plain yoghurt.

DID YOU KNOW?
Wheatberries are the most nutritious form of wheat, having both the bran and the germ, meaning maximum vitamins, minerals and fibre.

TASTY TIP
You can cook up a few extra wheatberries and sling them on a salad too. They'll keep in the fridge for 2–3 days.

Kedgeree-Do

Long before the Bhangra Beat, there was quite a carry on up the Khyber about a dish called 'khichri', made of rice and lentils. Adapted by the old Colonials into 'kedgeree' with fish and eggs, it's delicious and probably the Eighth Wonder of the World.

Serves 4

120 g/4 oz wholegrain rice
120 g/4 oz fresh haddock
225 g/8 oz smoked haddock
2 teaspoons curry powder
2 eggs, hard boiled
freshly ground black pepper

1   Cook the rice according to the instructions on the packet and leave to cool.

2   Now cook the fish. Put the fresh and smoked fish into 2 separate saucepans, add a little water and a teaspoon of curry powder over each, bring to the boil, then simmer. When cooked (5–10 minutes), pour the water away and flake the fish.

3   Slice the eggs or chop them into wedges.

4   Mix the rice and fish in a pan, season with the pepper, heat through, then put them in a dish and place the egg on top.

OUT OF THE KITCHEN AND INTO THE BATHROOM

Indian women are a dab hand at making their own beauty preparations. A popular cleanser is made from chickpea flour, ground lentils and a few herbs. Milk is added for dry skin and lemon juice for oily.

The Cholesterol Get Losterol Breakfast

Ask most Brits what they'd really like to wake up to in the morning (excluding Gaby's smile) and they'll say good old bacon and eggs. You're not denied that pleasure on the *Big Breakfast* diet, but the conditions are (1) no more than once a week and (2) it's got to be done in the most fat-sparingly way possible. So that means:

ıoı   GRILLING the bacon, mushrooms and tomatoes, rather than frying them.

ıoı   Saying SO LONG to sausages. But you could check out lower-fat sausages from time to time if you're really blue for bangers.

🍳 Frying the eggs in a non-stick pan with AS LITTLE BUT-TER AS POSSIBLE. Or, better still, POACHING them.

🍳 TOASTING the bread, not frying it.

🍳 If you have baked beans, make sure they're the LOW-SUGAR variety.

DID YOU KNOW?

that if you didn't have any conditioner, you could conditionyour hair with whisked egg. Rinse it out with cold orlukewarm water, though, otherwise it may scramble!

Our Daily Bread

There are bound to be days when you don't have time for a proper breakfast. But you know better than to skip it altogether. The basic ingredients for this breakfast are 2 slices of bread (preferably wholemeal, or at least granary) and 1 piece of fruit.

You could:

☕ Toast the bread and spread a little butter or low-fat spread on it, plus some honey or sugar-free jam. Munch it while you're getting ready or eat it on the way to work. Put an apple, orange or banana in your bag or pocket for later.

☕ Make a sandwich, say with a banana, some low-fat cream cheese, cottage cheese, Marmite or lean ham and take it with you. Don't forget the fruit if you haven't put it in your sandwich.

The Morning-After-the-Night-Before Breakfast

Your head feels like you've gone twelve rounds with Frank Bruno, a dripping tap sounds like Niagara Falls and your stomach is break-dancing. You vow you'll never drink again and you can't face food because you know five minutes later you'll be redecorating the walls with it. Time for a liquid breakfast that will do great shakes for the way you feel.

1 banana, mashed
juice of 2–3 oranges
2 tablespoons plain yoghurt
plus, if you want, a peach, a pear or a handful of
*   strawberries*

1   Blend and sip slowly with an aspirin or paracetamol tablet.

DID YOU KNOW?
Puerto Ricans claim to cure hangovers by rubbing lemon and lime juice into their armpits.

Flat as a Pancake

If at times you feel the only thing that's flat is your hair, try these tummy-tightening, posterior-pinching pancakes. Guaranteed to put life and bounce into your day.

Serves 4 people, 2 pancakes each

120 g/4 oz 81 per cent plain brown or wholemeal flour
a pinch of salt
1 egg
300 ml/½ pint skimmed milk (if using wholemeal flour
  you may need a little more)
1 teaspoon sunflower oil
a little sunflower oil or butter, for frying

1   Blend and sift the flour and salt into a bowl.

2   Beat the egg, milk and oil together, then add it slowly to the flour. Stir the mixture until you have a smooth batter.

3   Leave it to stand for about 20 minutes, then mix it all up again to ensure pancake perfection.

4   If you've got a good non-stick pan you might be able to get away with not using oil to fry the pancakes. Otherwise, use a minimal amount of sunflower oil or butter. When it's hot put in a couple of tablespoons of the pancake mixture and shake the pan so it spreads.

5   Cook the pancake for a couple of minutes on this side, flip it and cook the other side.

6   Keep the pancake warm in the oven while you cook the rest – you can stack them one on top of the other.

On your pancake try:

- a tablespoon of fruity sugar-free or sugar-reduced jam, spread all over and topped with a tablespoon of plain yoghurt
- chopped-up fresh fruit
- chopped-up apple, raisins and cinnamon
- cottage cheese

iOi   low-fat cream cheese

iOi   chocolate sauce and syrups *get the red card*

Nursery Rhyme Breakfast

> 'All the king's horses and all the king's men
> Couldn't put Humpty together again.'

Here's an old favourite starring soldiers that won't make a dumpy old Humpty out of you.

1   Boil 1 free-range egg for 4 minutes, so the white is cooked but the yolk is runny.

2   Toast 2 slices of brown bread, then thinly spread them with butter or low-fat spread. Cut 1 into soldiers and spread the other with Marmite or, if you don't like Marmite (how couldn't you?), with sugar-free jam, honey, or just leave it plain.

3   Dip away!

NB A word of warning: Small children, pregnant women, the sick and the elderly should always have their eggs hard-boiled.

The Go-Faster Breakfast

Warning: this breakfast isn't just called Go-Faster because it gives you energy. It really does make you get up and go!

Serves 4

Do your bowels a favour with:

450 g/1 lb mixed dried fruit (the average pre-packed
bag will contain apple rings, peaches, pears, prunes
and apricots)
1 carton unsweetened orange juice
plain yoghurt, low-fat crème fraîche or fromage frais,
to serve

1 Wash the fruit thoroughly under cool running water.

2 Put it in a bowl and pour over enough orange juice so it's covered. Leave to soak overnight.

3 Put the fruit and juice in a pan (you may need to add some water if the liquid has all but disappeared). Bring to the boil, then simmer for 10 minutes.

4 Serve hot or cold with a couple of tablespoons per person of plain yoghurt, low-fat crème fraîche (soured cream, like cream but less fattening) or plain fromage frais.

5 Join the queue for the bathroom.

WHERE IN THE WORLD . . .
would you find a fire engine on your plate for break-fast? In the Bahamas, that's where. It's corned beef, cooked with tomato paste and served up with grits, a kind of meal derived from corn.

WHAT'S ON THE BOX?

As well as all the suggestions here, your Big Breakfast could come out of a packet. Snap, cackle and . . . wait a minute . . .

Hooray: many ready-made breakfast cereals are for-tified with extra vitamins and minerals. But . . .

Boo: lots of them are also steeped in sugar – a sweet kiss of death to your diet. Before you buy, check the label for added sugar. And remember that the higher up the list of ingredients it appears, the more of it there is. Try to buy either sugar-free cereals or those that have reduced or little sugar. Good choices include Shredded Wheat, Grape Nuts, No Added Sugar Alpen, Jordan's Special Recipe Muesli, Puffed Wheat and Ready Brek.

In the bowl, zap cereals up with a chopped banana, chopped apple or handful of berries. And don't forget to use skimmed milk (or plain yoghurt).

The Macrobiotic Big Breakfast

How's your yang today? Yin and yang come from Chinese medicine and are opposite forces in nature. You think that's far out? There's more. Yang food tends to be more strength-ening and warming, while yin food is cooling. To best balance your yin and yang, natural, unprocessed and organic foods, high in complex carbohydrates and low in saturated fats, are recommended. Everyone can use yin and yang for breakfast – try the yang breakfast if you're feeling knackered and the yin one if you're feeling stressed out. Natural food experts Stephen and Jan Mosbacher, who gave us the recipes, swear by them.

Yang Breakfast: Vegetable Miso Soup

Serves 2

450 ml/15 fl. oz water
1 onion, cut in half moons
1 carrot, cut into matchsticks
7½-cm/3-inch piece of wakame sea vegetable (available in Japanese shops and many health food stores), soaked until tender then chopped
2 teaspoons miso (made from fermented soya bean; a delicious, but quite salty flavour. Available from most health food shops)
1 spring onion, finely chopped, for garnish

1   Put the water in a saucepan, add the onion and bring to the boil. Simmer for 2 minutes.
2   Add the carrot and wakame and simmer for 10 minutes.
3   Purée the miso with a little of the soup liquid and then add it to the soup.
4   Simmer for 2 minutes and garnish with the spring onion.
5   Serve with organic wholewheat bread, peanut butter and sauerkraut.

Yin Breakfast: Oatflake Porridge with Raisins and Soymilk

Serves 2

450 ml/15 fl. oz water
100 ml/4 oz oatflakes
a handful of raisins
a pinch of sea salt
150 ml/5 fl. oz soymilk

1 Put the water and oatflakes in a saucepan and bring to the boil.
2 Stir in the oatflakes, raisins and salt, then simmer for 10–20 minutes, stirring occasionally.
3 Add the soymilk, stir and simmer for a few more minutes.
4 Serve with a cup of herbal tea.

WHERE IN THE WORLD . . .
would you eat 'pho' for breakfast? In Vietnam, that's where. It's an aniseed-scented beef broth with noodles. Yum yum.

PARLEZ-VOUS
Seems these foreigners have got their breakfast all confused. In France, it's called 'petit déjeuner' or little lunch. Don't they know it's breakfast that's supposed to be bigger?

Sunday Brunch Apple Marmalade Pancakes

Super-healthy cook Jane Southern prepares food for the supermodels when they're being photographed for glossy magazines in London. This recipe's absolutely fabulous (without the champagne).

Serves 2–3

Pancake Mix

120 g/4 oz brown rice flour (available from health food shops) or 80 per cent wholemeal flour
50 g/2 oz rolled oats
a pinch of sea salt
1 teaspoon safflower oil
300 ml/½ pint apple juice
safflower oil, for frying

Mmmm Marmalade

225 ml/8 fl. oz apple juice
100 ml/4 fl. oz orange juice
450 g/1 lb cooking apples, peeled and grated
1 orange, chopped
½ teaspoon sea salt
rind of 1 orange, cut into very thin strips
50 g/2 oz barley malt, rice syrup or maple syrup
2 teaspoons fresh ginger juice (grate fresh ginger and squeeze out juices)

1   To make the pancakes: mix the flour and oats. Add the salt, the oil and apple juice and mix into a batter. Set aside for 20 minutes.

2 Heat a non-stick frying pan, brush lightly with oil and ladle in enough batter to cover the base. Cook until holes appear, then turn over and brown lightly. Serve with the apple marmalade, made this way . . .

3 Put the apple and orange juices into a saucepan and add the apple, orange and salt. Bring to the boil, cover and simmer for 5–10 minutes.

4 Meanwhile, cover the orange rind with water and bring to the boil. Throw away the water and repeat.

Films with a breakfast connection:

☞ *Breakfast at Tiffany's*
☞ *The Breakfast Club*
☞ Er . . .

EGGSTRA, EGGSTRA, READ ALL ABOUT IT

Eggs are good for you, but do contain fat and the yolk has lots of dietary cholesterol. Aim to eat about four a week and no more than six. Don't put all your eggs in one basket, though – check that you're not getting eggstra in ready-prepared dishes.

There's an eggciting idea from America around at the moment – the yolkless scrambled egg breakfast. We think scrambled eggs without the yolk taste totally terrible. Why bother, and what do you do with the yolks anyway? Our advice: if you want scrambled eggs, cook them in a non-stick pan so you don't have to use extra fat.

5   Now combine the rind with the barley malt and simmer
until it is absorbed.

6   Remove half of the apple and orange mixture and
purée it. Return it to the saucepan, add the ginger juice
and simmer till thick.

7   Stir in the sweetened rind and serve with the pancakes.
If there's marmalade left over, have it on your toast.

HONEY, YOUR SKIN IS SO SOFT

*Here's a handy little DIY face-mask you can whisk up in
your kitchen. It's great for normal to dry skin. Mix 1
tablespoon honey with 2 tablespoons oatmeal and
make into a paste. Spread it all over your face and
neck. Leave on for 15 minutes then lick, sorry,* rinse *it
off.*

Big Bad Breakfasts

These items are NOT on the menu . . .

☕ Chocolate chip muffins, Danish pastries, plain and
filled croissants.

☕ Sausage and bacon sandwiches with so much butter
that the fat's running down your chin and arms, then
making a quick sprint for your hips.

- ☕ Sugar-coated cereals with an extra 3 spoonfuls of sugar on top.
- ☕ Anything with full-fat milk. Think skim and slim.
- ☕ A loaf of white bread, toasted and topped with chocolate spread, lemon curd and any other gooey, syrupy, very sweet things.
- ☕ Daily fried bacon, eggs, black pudding, sausages, bread, baked beans, mushrooms and tomatoes. See the Cholesterol Get Losterol Breakfast (page 44) for the safer-for-slimmers version.

CHAPTER FOUR

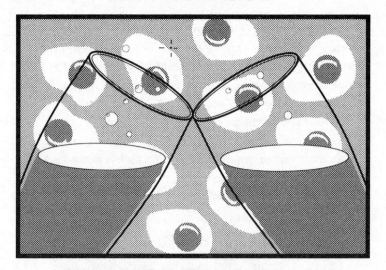

Let's Do Lunch . . .

If you can lunch like a prince, i.e. have a good cooked one, that's ideal. Cooking your own puts you in control. If you rely on a canteen, check the recipes here for the kind of things you should be choosing and if they're not available show them this book. If you're office-bound, there are probably local sandwich bars that offer, at the very least, baked potatoes.

It Hasta Be Pasta or a Spud

The humble baked potato is a secret powerhouse packed with all sorts of nutritious niceness, including vitamin C. There's plenty of fibre in it too, ensuring you don't get all blocked up. Pasta is another magic food, high in carbo-hydrate, and if you choose the unrefined (wholewheat) ver-sions you get extra Brownie points because they're a lot better for you. With pasta, take 2–3 tablespoons (uncooked) as an average serving.

What's nice on pasta is nice in a baked potato too! Dieters should avoid creamy, buttery, fattening sauces and be led from the temptation to drown a jacket potato in a sea of butter. Try the following fillings and toppings, all based on serving two.

Sweetcorn and Red Pepper

1   Sweat a small chopped onion and a chopped clove of garlic in 1 tablespoon olive or sunflower oil. To sweat means to lightly 'fry' in a little oil on a low heat, so the onion softens slightly and turns a bit 'sweaty'-looking.

2   When sweated, add 1 chopped red pepper (de-seeded) and stir occasionally.

3   After 5 minutes, add about 120 g/4 oz of sweetcorn (either frozen or from a tin – but make sure there's no added sugar). Heat through, season with freshly ground black pepper and fresh herbs and mix in 1 tablespoon low-fat crème fraîche (which gives a creamy texture, minus the calories of cream).

Mushroom

1   Start, as above, by sweating a chopped onion and chopped clove of garlic. Add 250 g/9 oz sliced fresh mushrooms and season.

2 If you're going to use this topping for a baked potato, add 1 tablespoon of low-fat crème fraîche or plain yoghurt. For pasta, serve it topped with 50 g/2 oz of grated low-fat Cheddar.

3 Chopped parsley sprinkled over makes it extra yummy.

Bolognese

1 Dry fry (i.e. without oil on a low heat) 120 g/4 oz of the leanest mince you can buy. When the juices start running, add 1 chopped onion and 1–2 cloves of chopped garlic, 1 very finely chopped carrot and 1 chopped celery stalk.

2 Keep stirring for about 15 minutes, then add a small tin of tomatoes and black pepper, plus some oregano or herbs de Provence (about ½ teaspoon each).

3 Simmer on a low heat, stirring occasionally, for about 20 minutes. Finish off with 1 tablespoon low-fat crème fraîche or plain yoghurt.

Vegetable Bolognese

1 Again begin by sweating your chopped onion and garlic clove.

2 Then add 1 teaspoon finely chopped or grated ginger, 1 finely chopped carrot, 1 chopped celery stalk and, if you want, half a bulb of chopped fennel.

3 Turn the mixture around over the heat for about 5 minutes, add a small tin of chopped tomatoes and 80 g/3 oz split red lentils (washed) and any herbs you like.

4 Bring to the boil, then simmer for 20–25 minutes. You

might have to add a couple of tablespoons of water. Finish with 1 tablespoon of low-fat crème fraîche or plain yoghurt and some chopped parsley.

Tuna

1   Start as described above with your onion and garlic.
2   Add a small tin of chopped tomatoes, seasoning, herbs and 1 teaspoon lemon juice. Simmer for about 10 minutes.
3   Drain a 200-g/7-oz tin of tuna (in brine or water, not oil) and break the chunks up a bit. Add them to the sauce and heat through.

Cheese and Herb

1   Start with your onion and garlic as before.
2   Mash 200 g/7 oz low-fat cream cheese with 3 table-spoons herbs (e.g. parsley, dill, chives – whatever you fancy) and melt in the onion mixture.
3   Add the juice of 1 small lemon, a dash of Worcester-shire sauce, and voilà!

Spinach

1   Sweat a chopped onion and clove of garlic in 1 table-spoon oil, as described above.
2   Add 300 g/11 oz frozen leaf spinach. Thaw over a low heat for about 10 minutes. Season with black pepper and some grated nutmeg and serve with 50 g/2 oz grated low-fat cheese on top.

Rainbow Vegetables

This is best cooked in a non-stick wok, though you can do it in a large non-stick pan.

1　Wash and chop a 250-g/10-oz selection of vegetables. For example, 50 g/2 oz broccoli, 50 g/2 oz carrots, 50 g/2 oz red pepper, 50 g/2 oz cauliflower and 50 g/ 2 oz mangetout. Many supermarkets now sell baby vegetables, which don't need chopping up. Whichever veggies you choose, go for a bright, colourful selection, as much for visual interest as the different tastes.

2　Start by sweating 1 small chopped onion and a chopped clove of garlic in 1 tablespoon oil. When they're glossy, start to add the vegetables, the hardest first as they take longest to cook.

3　Keep stirring the vegetables – you may need to add a few drops of water. You can also add 1 teaspoon chopped or grated ginger if you like the taste. Flavour with a dash of interesting sauce, such as soy or sweet and sour, and cook to your preferred level of vegetable crispness.

Prawns with Garlic and Piri Piri

This is probably nicer with pasta than it is in a baked potato. See what you think.

1　Start by sweating the chopped onion and, this time, 2–3 chopped cloves of garlic, in oil.

2　Add 1 finely chopped and de-seeded chilli pepper and cook for a couple of minutes. Then add a generous pinch of piri piri (a hot spice you can now find in most supermarkets) or chilli powder. You may need to add a little more oil or water.

3 Now mix in 200 g/7 oz defrosted prawns. Heat through, stirring frequently.

4 Finish off by adding a couple of tablespoons chopped fresh herbs, such as coriander, dill and parsley.

Rice 'n' Easy!

Apart from serving rice with 'saucy' dishes (you could put the potato and pasta toppings on a steaming bed of it), you can also combine it in the pot with vegetables, pulses, seafood, fish, meat, seeds, or a combination of these, to make a dish of its own. Rice is nice because:

- ιοι it contains protein, iron, zinc and some B vitamins, as well as carbohydrate
- ιοι it's high in fibre and fills you up without fattening you up
- ιοι experts say grains are one of the foods we should be eating more of

Don't get in a paddy, though – here are some ideas for what to do with it.

Rice Up

You need about 50 g/2 oz (uncooked weight) per person. You can up the quantity by an ounce or two for non-dieters. Always rinse the rice under cold running water first to clean it.

1 Instead of plain boiling, you might like to try something a little more interesting. Chop an onion and 1–2 cloves of garlic. You could also chop up any other hard veg you might want to use, such as carrots or fennel. Throw the onions, garlic and veg in the pot and 'sweat' them in 1 tablespoon olive or sunflower oil over a very low heat, so they soften up a bit and go glossy.

2   Add the rice and stir. Now add around 4–5 fl. oz or 100–150 ml of stock or water per person, i.e. per 50 g/ 2 oz rice, and season. To tickle the tastebuds, experiment with seasonings such as cumin, coriander, allspice, turmeric, chilli powder, curry powder or simply some fresh herbs. You could also add lentils at this stage (25 g/1 oz per person). Bring to the boil, stir, then turn down the heat, simmering for about 30 minutes.

3   Add any other softer vegetables, such as peppers or mushrooms, about 10 minutes before the end of cooking. You could also throw in some greens at this stage, or you could steam them separately.

4   Serve this tasty lot with a sprinkling of grated low-fat cheese – only an ounce or two for slimmers, mind.

ιοι   PRAWN COCKTAIL. If using frozen prawns, make sure you defrost them thoroughly and add them in the final minutes of cooking.

ιοι   A FISHY TALE. Raw fish needs cubing and putting in about 5–10 minutes before you finish cooking.

ιοι   MEATHEAD. If you want to use up left-over meat, cut it very fine or shred it and make sure it's cooked through thoroughly.

ιοι   For the adventurous tastebud, you could include some chopped ready-to-eat dried apricots (when you start cooking the rice), as well as a few pumpkin or sunflower seeds and/or flaked almonds (10 minutes before the end of cooking).

Delicious Dishes with Fishes

Fish cookery is an art and this isn't a Delia Smith cook book, but here are some healthy, diet-conscious ways with which to experiment. Fish is always fintastic served with vegetables or salad, rice or potatoes. If it's saucy, it's great with pasta too.

A Serious Grilling

1   You can grill whole fish (not too big) or fish steaks (not too thick). Try marinating them first for a couple of hours in a little olive or sunflower oil with lemon juice, herbs, garlic and black pepper. If time is too short to do this, just brush them lightly with the same mixture before grilling. For extra flavour you can also stuff a whole fish with herbs and a clove of garlic. Sardines and mackerel don't need any extra oil – they're what you might call slippery customers.

2   Preheat the grill to a medium temperature and don't put the fish too close to the heat to begin with – this way you'll avoid excessive browning. Cooking time depends on the size of the fish – let 'Observe and Prod' be your watchword.

Doing the Billingsgate Bake

1 Baking is fab for a whole fish. Start by marinating it in some oil and herbs for a couple of hours in an oven-proof dish, turning frequently.

2 Surround the fish with sliced onions, a clove or two of garlic, chopped tomato and maybe some celery or fennel, before putting it in a medium-hot oven (180–200°C/350–400°F/Gas Mark 4–6) – the bigger the fish the hotter the oven should be.

3 Baste frequently with lime or lemon juice, and near the end of cooking, scoop up the cooking juices for basting. (Isn't 'baste' a good word?)

TICK TOCK: as a rough guide, 1 kg/2 lb fish requires 30 to 40 minutes' cooking time.

It's a Wrap

Try this with fish steaks, cutlets or slices.

1 First prepare the flavourings. Finely chop whatever you choose to put in your parcel: for example, ginger, onions, spring onions, apple, mushrooms, peppers, chilli peppers, garlic and herbs (dill, coriander and parsley are particularly good for fish).

2 Cut foil to fit loosely around your fish then put the fish in the centre. Add your extra bits, moisten with lemon or lime juice and wrap it all up well, but leave some air space.

3 Preheat the oven to 180°C/350°F/Gas Mark 4, and cook according to size – about 10 minutes for a 120-g/4-oz steak.

Top of the Stove

This way's good for cod or similar fillets.

On a bed of tomatoes and onions:

1 Chop 1–2 onions and 1–2 cloves of garlic. Dry fry or sweat them slowly in 1 tablespoon oil.

2 Add a medium-sized tin of chopped tomatoes, black pepper and herbs.

3 Let the mixture simmer for about 15 minutes, then put the fish on top and steam it on the bed for about 5 minutes or until cooked.

On a bed of onion, pepper and potato:

1 Sweat the onion and garlic as above. Then add a chopped red pepper, a finely chopped chilli pepper (optional) and 2 chopped tomatoes.

2 Now add 2 small to medium-sized potatoes (quartered if necessary) per person, a pinch of chilli powder, or curry powder if you like, a little chopped parsley, black pepper and chopped coriander.

3 Add a minimum of 200 ml/⅓ pint (depending on how many potatoes you are cooking) veg or fish stock.

4 Cook for 20 minutes or until the potatoes are nearly done. Add the fish and give it another 5–10 minutes, depending on its size.

Count Your Chickens

Chicken is a good source of low-fat protein. The important thing to remember, though, is that the skin contains most of the fat, so it should be removed. It's a very versatile food – easy to dress up (have you ever seen a chicken in a tuxedo and tiara?), great just plain grilled and is as yummy cold as it is hot.

Braise Be!

To braise chicken – dry fry or sauté it in very little oil, say a tablespoon or less, before adding liquid, such as vegetable or chicken stock or orange juice. Then add a variety of luscious things like apples, dried fruit, almonds, small whole onions and/or peppers, tomatoes, olives, pineapple, oranges and kiwi. Then just simmer till tender.

Out of the Frying Pan into the Grill

For grilling, get creative with seasoning to make it more interesting.

- ⦿ Exotic, Eastern-inspired flavours include lemon juice and/or ginger, curry powder or paste, cayenne pepper, and soy sauce. *Ah so!*

- ⦿ Mediterranean-style flavours include the herbs thyme, oregano, rosemary and ready-mixed selections such as herbs de Provence. Garlic is, of course, not to be forgotten! *Ciao bella!*

The Sunday Roast

In the *Big Breakfast* diet, roasting is allowed too (yippee!). But – there had to be a but, didn't there? – it's got to be done without fat. If you can spit roast, that's brilliant.

1 Stuff the chicken with tarragon, rub the skin with salt, pepper and paprika, and pour a little cold water (say 5 tablespoons) over and around the bird.

2 Put it in the oven at 200°C/400°F/Gas Mark 6 for not less than 1 hour. Before eating remove all the skin.

3 Eat 1 breast or 1 leg, hot, with lots of vegetables, plus rice or potatoes (no roasted ones, if you're being strict about dieting; OK if you've reached your target weight and they're just for a treat). If served cold, have the chicken with lots of salad, plus a baked potato, or in a more interesting salad – see Chapter 5.

To Be or Nut To Be

Serves 4 nutters

120 g/4 oz hazelnuts, finely chopped
120 g/4 oz almonds, finely chopped
225 g/8 oz tomatoes, skinned, de-seeded and diced
1 medium-sized onion, diced
½ green or red pepper, diced
1 small clove of garlic, chopped
1 teaspoon mild curry powder
2 eggs, beaten

1 Preheat the oven to 180°C/350°F/Gas Mark 4.

2 Place the chopped nuts in a bowl with the tomatoes, onion, pepper, garlic and curry powder.

3 Stir in the beaten eggs and mix the whole lot together thoroughly. Spoon the mixture into a 1-kg/2-lb loaf tin or 23-cm/8-inch square cake tin.

4 Bake for 20–30 minutes until firm. Serve with a large mixed salad or plenty of vegetables. And if the person sitting next to you takes too much, nut them.

Zig and Zag's Bake

This one's a favourite in Zog where Zig and Zag come from.

Serves 4 Zoggians

225 g/8 oz pasta shells (preferably wholewheat)
350 g/12 oz cauliflower florets or 1 small cauliflower
1 small onion, diced
1 clove of garlic, crushed
1 small leek, finely chopped
1 teaspoon dried mixed herbs
5 tablespoons dry white wine (optional)
1 × 200-g/7-oz tin chopped tomatoes (choose one with
  no added sugar or salt)
75 g/ 3 oz low-fat Cheddar cheese
a pinch of salt and black pepper

1 Preheat the oven to 190°C/375°F/Gas Mark 5.
2 Cook the pasta according to instructions on the packet, then drain. Steam the cauliflower until just tender.
3 In a medium-sized saucepan, gently dry fry the onion, garlic, leek and mixed herbs for a couple of minutes. Add the wine (or substitute water) and cook for another 2 minutes.
4 Pour in the tomatoes and simmer for 15–20 minutes until the sauce has thickened and reduced slightly. Season with salt and pepper.

5 Fold in the cooked pasta and cauliflower and spoon the mixture into an ovenproof dish.

6 Sprinkle the cheese on top and cook for 15 minutes or until golden brown.

Zoggians serve this one with extra vegetables, such as broccoli (or a local favourite, Ziggymondius, available from all good Zoggian supermarkets).

Pizza Express

Grab a pizza de action with this 'I can't believe it's not junk food' recipe.

Serves 4 Italians

225 g/8 oz plain wholemeal flour
½ teaspoon baking powder
50 g/2 oz low-fat spread
50 g/2 oz chopped tomatoes, drained
1 small clove of garlic, chopped
½ small onion, diced
2 rashers lean bacon, grilled and diced
120 g/4 oz button mushrooms, sliced
½ teaspoon dried mixed herbs
120 g/4 oz half-fat cheese, such as Shape
freshly ground black pepper

1 Make the base: using a fork, work together the flour, baking powder and low-fat spread. Slowly add enough water to form a soft dough. Cover and allow to rest for 1 hour in the fridge.

2   Preheat the oven to 200°C/400°F/Gas Mark 6.

3   Roll out the dough to form a 20-cm/8-inch circle. Transfer to a non-stick baking tray and cook for 10 minutes.

4   Spread the tomatoes and remaining ingredients over the base, finishing with a sprinkling of black pepper and the cheese. Put it back into the oven and cook for 10–15 minutes or until golden brown.

5   Serve hot or cold, with a salad.

Lock-Keeper's Mackerel

Cook this up in the kitchen and you won't have to fish for compliments – they'll fall for it hook, line and sinker.

Serves 4 lock-keepers

1 small onion, diced
1 small carrot, diced
1 tablespoon plain flour
1 × 400-g/14-oz can tomatoes
2 teaspoons tomato purée
300 ml/½ pint fish stock
1 clove of garlic, chopped
1 bay leaf, crumbled
4 × 120-g/4-oz fresh mackerel fillets
50 g/2 oz black olives, pitted and sliced
freshly ground black pepper
fresh basil, to garnish

1   In a non-stick frying pan, dry fry the onion and carrot for a couple of minutes. Sprinkle on the flour and stir for a further minute.

2 Add the tomatoes, purée, stock, garlic and bay leaf. Bring to the boil, then reduce the heat and simmer for 35–45 minutes.

3 Liquidize or purée the sauce, then sieve into a small pan and keep warm.

4 Cut each mackerel fillet in half lengthwise and steam (in a steamer) for 7–10 minutes or until cooked (or you could grill them).

5 Transfer the fish to the serving plate. Stir the black olives into the sauce and season with black pepper, then spoon it over the fish. Garnish with basil.

6 Serve with brown rice or small boiled potatoes and a selection of vegetables.

Chicken Chegwin

Serves 4 early-morning risers in Leicester

4 × 150-g/5-oz boneless chicken breasts
1 onion, diced
1 clove of garlic, crushed
120 g/4 oz tomatoes, skinned, de-seeded and
  chopped
120 g/4 oz mushrooms, thickly sliced
2 sprigs fresh tarragon, chopped
1 teaspoon tomato purée
600 ml/1 pint chicken stock
freshly ground black pepper

1 Preheat the oven to 190°C/375°F/Gas Mark 5.

2 Place the chicken breasts in an ovenproof dish and

cook for 7 minutes, to seal the chicken. Remove the skin at this stage, if you haven't already done so.

3   Dry fry the onion and garlic until softened, then add the tomatoes, mushrooms, tarragon and tomato purée. Simmer for a few minutes, then stir in the chicken stock.

4   Pour the sauce over the chicken breasts, cover and cook in the oven for a further 20 minutes or until the chicken is tender. Season with black pepper.

Dish the Fish

Serves 1 (2 would be unfair on the salmon)

1 × 120–150 g/4–5 oz salmon steak
1–2 tablespoons water
1 tablespoon wholegrain mustard
1 teaspoon paprika
a few drops tabasco sauce

1   Lay the salmon in a small ovenproof dish.

2   Mix the rest of the ingredients together and pour over the fish.

3   Place at the top of a preheated oven (220°C/425°F/Gas Mark 7) for 5 minutes or until the fish is cooked to your taste.

4   Pour off the mixture before serving so the fish is just slightly flavoured.

5   Serve with vegetables and new potatoes or brown rice, or a mixed salad.

Fish of the Day

Serves 2 cod-tented citizens

1 small red pepper, de-seeded and chopped
1 small onion, chopped
1 small tin tomatoes
½ teaspoon chilli powder
½ teaspoon paprika
1 clove of garlic, crushed
120 g/4 oz rice
½ teaspoon turmeric (optional)
2 courgettes
2 pieces cod, around 150 g/5 oz each in size

1 Put all the ingredients except the rice, turmeric, courgettes and fish into a saucepan and bring to the boil. Then simmer gently on a reduced heat for 15 minutes.

2 Liquidize until smooth, and keep warm.

3 Cook the rice, with the turmeric, according to the instructions on the packet.

4 Grate the courgettes lengthwise and add them to the rice.

5 Meanwhile grill the fish for around 4 minutes on each side or until cooked.

6 Pour the sauce over the fish and serve with the rice and courgettes.

Lean-i Fettuccini

Serves 4 who lean towards cottage cheese
(some people do, OK. Live and let live)

120 g/4 oz low-fat plain yoghurt
120 g/4 oz low-fat cottage cheese
2–3 cloves of garlic, finely chopped
½ tablespoon lemon zest
a pinch of freshly ground black pepper
350 g/12 oz dried fettuccini pasta
2 tablespoons fresh parsley, chopped
25 g/1 oz Parmesan cheese

1   Combine the yoghurt, cottage cheese, garlic, lemon zest and black pepper in a blender and blend until creamy. Set aside.

2   Cook the pasta according to the instructions on the packet, then drain in a bowl and toss with the parsley and Parmesan.

3   Add the creamy mixture and toss again.

4   Serve with a mixed salad.

5   Now call the nearest travel agent and book a fortnight in Tuscany.

Bikini-Friendly Blinis

Serves 4 tanned and happy beach bodies

85 g/3¼ oz brown lentils
200 ml/⅓ pint vegetable stock
2 tablespoons sherry vinegar
1 tablespoon tomato purée
250 g/9 oz potatoes, peeled and cubed
1 chilli pepper, finely chopped
1 walnut-sized piece of fresh ginger, finely chopped
a few spring onions, finely chopped
sunflower or olive oil, for brushing
450 g/1 lb eating apples or 300 g/11 oz ready-to-eat
   dried apricots
1 tablespoon lemon juice
4 tablespoons orange juice

1 Cook the lentils in the stock and vinegar for 10 minutes on a high heat then 20 minutes on a low heat. Add the tomato purée.

2 Cook the potatoes for 12–15 minutes, drain and mash them.

3 Mix the chilli, ginger, spring onions and lentils into the mashed potato.

4 Line a baking tray with foil or baking parchment and heat the oven to 200°C/400°F/Gas Mark 6. To make 8 blinis, put 8 tablespoons of the mixture on different parts of the tray and flatten them. Brush with the tiniest amount of oil and bake for 15 minutes.

5 Wash and chop the apples (or apricots) and marinate

in the fruit juices. Pour this over the blinis when they're cooked.

Fill It with Millet

Feeds 2 milletants

You'll find millet in all health food stores and many super-markets. It's got more protein and iron than other grains (so it's especially good for vegetarians), it's cheap and it fills you up. It's also gluten-free – good for folks with gluten allergies.

120 g/4 oz millet
600 ml/1 pint vegetable stock
150 g/5 oz Edam or Gouda cheese, grated
1 leek, finely chopped
1 whole egg
1 egg yolk
1 teaspoon oil
salt and freshly ground pepper
a little lemon juice
500 g/1 lb tomatoes, chopped

1 Preheat the oven to 200°C/400°F/Gas Mark 6.
2 In a large strainer rinse the millet with boiling water, then cook it in the stock for about 30 minutes on a low heat (all the liquid should disappear).
3 Add the cheese and leek to the millet with the egg and yolk and season with a little salt and pepper and lemon juice.
4 Put in a lightly greased flat Pyrex dish.

5   Bake in the oven for 15 minutes.
6   Make a dressing from the lemon juice, salt and pepper and pour over the tomatoes.

Blow-Your-Socks-Off Chilli

Serves 2 Mexicans

1 onion, finely chopped
2 cloves of garlic, finely chopped
1 tablespoon olive oil
2 carrots, sliced
2 celery sticks, chopped into small chunks
1 apple, diced
chilli powder
1 small tin chopped tomatoes
1 small tin kidney beans
1 green pepper, diced
120 g/4 oz mushrooms, whole or sliced
2 small courgettes, sliced
120 g/4 oz frozen peas
120 g/4 oz tinned or frozen sweetcorn
salt/pepper
½ teaspoon dried mixed herbs or oregano

1   Sweat the onion and garlic in the oil.
2   After a few minutes add the carrots, celery and apple. Add the chilli powder – to your taste or, should we *say*, tolerance level – and stir over a very low heat (if you burn chilli powder it gets bitter).

3   Now add the tin of tomatoes and seasoning and simmer for 5 minutes.

4   Add the beans, green pepper and mushrooms. Stir and simmer for about 20 minutes.

5   Add the courgettes, peas and sweetcorn. Stir and cook for another few minutes.

6   Serve with brown rice.

Vegetarian Nirvana

Serves 2 Buddhists

80 g/3 oz millet
300 ml/½ pint vegetable stock
2 leeks, chopped into small rings
200 g/7 oz broccoli, broken into small florets
2 tablespoons olive or sunflower oil
salt
freshly ground black pepper or cayenne pepper
3 tablespoons low-fat crème fraîche
1 teaspoon lemon juice

1   Rinse the millet with boiling water and cook it in the vegetable stock for about 20 minutes.

2   Cook the leeks and broccoli in the oil, preferably in a wok.

3   Add the millet, season with salt and pepper (try cayenne). Add the crème fraîche and lemon juice.

CHAPTER FIVE

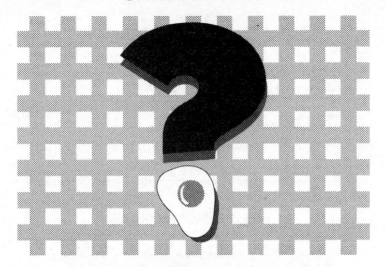

Guess What's for Dinner

Now it's time to dine like a pauper. Don't worry, it's not that bad. Just remember that on the *Big Breakfast* diet, dinner is your lightest meal, so try to choose it from this section, which is all about soups, salads and sandwiches.

Remember also to eat your dinner as early as you can to work some of it off before you go to bed.

You can have a soup, a salad and a sandwich, if you want. But, if you're going for a hat-trick, make the salad a simple mixed one, i.e. don't have one of the deluxe salads with lots of extra bits. Likewise you could have a soup and a sensational salad, say with pasta and chicken, but you'd have to compromise on the sandwich and just have two slices of bread without the filling. Get the picture? If you want a change you can also substitute a baked potato for a sandwich or throw a handful of cooked rice in your soup from time to time.

Try to eat this way, with the lighter dinner, if you want to follow the diet strictly. You can swap lunches and dinners around when, for one reason or another, it's not practical to follow the plan. And, if you find it really hard to eat this way during the week, do at least try to follow it at the weekend.

Don't forget that the recipes and principles in this book are also a way to a healthier lifestyle, so they work for non-dieters too.

Souped Up

There are lots of good commercially prepared soups on supermarket shelves. Go for the low-cal ones and those that don't have added cream or sugar. Better still, make your own.

Very Orange Soup

Serves 4

1 tablespoon olive oil
1 medium-sized onion, chopped
1 large carrot, chopped
1 medium-sized potato, cut into chunks

900 ml/1½ pints vegetable stock
juice of 1 orange
salt and pepper to taste

1   Heat the olive oil in a saucepan, throw the veggies in and toss them for a few minutes.
2   Next add the vegetable stock and simmer for 30 minutes or so until the vegetables are tender.
3   Let the mixture cool, then blend it in a liquidizer, adding the orange juice and seasoning, to taste.

Skinny Soup

Serves 4

1 kg/2¼ lb fresh tomatoes, roughly chopped
1 small onion, roughly chopped
1 small clove of garlic, finely chopped
50 g/2 oz carrots, roughly chopped
50 g/2 oz celery, roughly chopped
900 ml/1½ pints vegetable stock
10–15 basil leaves
1 dessertspoon tomato purée
½ teaspoon artificial sweetener, such as Canderel
salt and freshly ground black pepper, to taste

1   Put the tomatoes, onion, garlic, carrots and celery in a large saucepan with the stock, basil leaves, tomato purée and sweetener.
2   Bring to the boil, then cover and simmer for 20 minutes or so, until the veggies are soft.

3   Purée the mixture in a blender, then sieve it, add seasoning and serve up hot.

TIP: this soup is also nice served cold with some plain yoghurt swirled through it.

Magical Mushroom Soup

Serves 4

175 g/6 oz mushrooms, roughly chopped
120 g/4 oz onions, chopped
75 g/3 oz celery, chopped
½ teaspoon dried mixed herbs
600 ml/1 pint vegetable stock
300 ml/½ pint skimmed milk
freshly ground black pepper

1   Put the mushrooms in a large saucepan with the onion, celery, herbs and stock.
2   Bring to the boil, cover and simmer for 15–20 minutes.
3   Purée the mixture in a blender, then put it back in the pan, add the milk and bring back to the boil. Season with black pepper.

It-Won't-Show-on-the-Scales Minestrone

Serves 4

50 g/2 oz carrots, diced
50 g/2 oz onions, diced
50 g/2 oz celery, chopped
50 g/2 oz tomatoes, skinned and chopped
50 g/2 oz button mushrooms, diced
50 g/2 oz courgettes, diced
2 cloves of garlic, chopped
25 g/1 oz wholegrain pasta shells or macaroni
1 tablespoon tomato purée
1–2 teaspoons dried mixed herbs
1.2 litres/2 pints vegetable stock
freshly ground black pepper

1 Put all the vegetables into a big saucepan with the garlic, pasta, tomato purée, herbs and stock.

2 Bring to the boil, then cover and simmer for 15–20 minutes until the veggies are soft. Season with black pepper.

Salad Days

From simple mixed to mega-mix, salads *can* be interesting.
Trust us.

Dressing up the Salad

Lotta Yoghurt Dressing

225 ml/8 fl. oz low-fat plain yoghurt
100 ml/4 fl. oz skimmed milk
*2–3 tablespoons chopped fresh herbs (whatever you
    like)*
1 clove of garlic, crushed
1 teaspoon honey
salt and freshly ground black pepper, to taste

1   Whisk everything together by hand or let the blender
    take the strain.

The French Way

2 tablespoons olive oil
1 tablespoon cider vinegar or white wine vinegar
a pinch of freshly ground black pepper
½ teaspoon mustard
*2 tablespoons chopped fresh herbs or a pinch of dried
    mixed herbs*

1   Mix and whisk together! Ooo la la!

or try

ɪ○ɪ　just putting lemon juice on as a dressing

ɪ○ɪ　using plain yoghurt with plenty of herbs and onion

ɪ○ɪ　buying the lowest-cal dressing you can find – go easy
　　on the mayonnaise and salad cream

Pounds-Away Pasta

Serves 2–3

*225 g/8 oz pasta (anything but spaghetti, and
　preferably brown), cooked*
225 g/8 oz diced chicken breast, cooked
*50 g/2 oz each of tomatoes, green pepper, red pepper
　(or any other raw vegetable you like)*
plus, if you want, 25–50 g/1–2 oz onion, finely chopped

1　Just mix and serve! (See the dressing recipes above.)

Down Mexico Way

Serves 4

*275 g/10 oz mixed frozen vegetables – most
　supermarkets have the ready-diced sort with peas,
　beans, peppers, etc*
120 g/4 oz frozen (or tinned) sweetcorn
275 g/10 oz small frozen prawns, defrosted
2 tablespoons lemon juice
4 tablespoons olive oil

1 clove of garlic, finely chopped
a pinch of allspice
salt and freshly ground black pepper, to taste
1 lettuce

1 Cook the frozen veggies and the sweetcorn according to the instructions on the packet and leave them to cool.

2 Put the prawns in a large bowl and pour over the dressing made from the lemon juice, oil, garlic, allspice and salt and pepper.

3 Mix in the vegetables and serve on a bed of lettuce.

Goodness Greekcious

Serves 3

1 small lettuce, preferably Iceberg
150 g/5 oz cucumber, chopped
8 medium-sized tomatoes, chopped
225 g/8 oz Feta cheese, diced
4 basil leaves, torn
12 black olives

1 Tear up the lettuce and add the chopped cucumber and tomatoes, the diced Feta and the torn basil leaves.

2 Leave the olives whole or slice them and add to the salad. Pour on your choice of dressing.

3 Serve with pitta bread and a small amount of dip, such as taramasalata or hummus.

Name That Tuna

Serves 4

1 small lettuce (Cos, Iceberg, Frisée, or plain old
   English Garden, you choose)
1 × 200-g/7-oz tin tuna chunks in brine (dolphin-
   friendly, of course)
8 small tomatoes
150 g/5 oz cucumber
120 g/4 oz canned or frozen sweetcorn, cooked
150 g/5 oz cooked green beans or 1 small tin
   butterbeans or kidney beans
2 eggs, boiled and sliced
1 small onion, finely chopped
1 tablespoon fresh herbs, e.g. dill and/or parsley

1   Just chop, slice and mix it all up.

Totally Tropical Salad

Serves 4

225 g/8 oz rice (preferably wholegrain or basmati)
1 mango
4 slices fresh pineapple, or tinned (check there's no
   added sugar)
1 papaya
50 g/2 oz seedless grapes

*50 g/2 oz flaked almonds or 2 tablespoons sunflower
   or pumpkin seeds
3 tablespoons olive oil
2 tablespoons lemon juice
a pinch of ground cloves
salt and freshly ground black pepper, to taste*

1   Cook the rice according to the instructions on the packet.
    Drain and leave to cool.
2   Wash, peel and dice or slice the fruit.
3   Mix the rice, fruit and nuts or seeds together.
4   Make the dressing by mixing together the oil, lemon
    juice, cloves and seasoning. Add to the rice mixture and
    chill.

Tabbouleh to Go

Serves 4

*225 g/8 oz bulgur wheat (you can buy it in health
   food stores and most supermarkets)
1 bunch parsley, chopped
4–5 spring onions, chopped
8 medium-sized tomatoes, chopped
2 fresh mint leaves, finely chopped
4 tablespoons olive oil
3 tablespoons lemon juice
salt and freshly ground black pepper, to taste*

1   Soak the bulgur wheat in a bowl of cold water for 25–30
    minutes, until the grains swell up. Drain thoroughly.

2   Put the parsley, spring onions and tomatoes in a bowl with the wheat. Add the mint.

3   Make a dressing with the oil, lemon juice, salt and pepper and pour it over the salad. Toss and chill.

Slimline Smoked Mackerel Salad

Serves 4

275 g/10 oz pasta shapes (such as penne)
275 g/10 oz smoked mackerel fillets
1 tablespoon lemon juice
freshly ground black pepper
1 large apple, diced
1 bulb of fennel, diced
4 sticks of celery, chopped

1   Cook the pasta according to the instructions on the packet.

2   Flake the mackerel fillets and place them in a small bowl with the lemon juice and a sprinkling of black pepper.

3   Into this bowl add the pasta and remaining ingredients and mix together. Dress with French dressing or try:

150 ml/¼ pint low-cal mayonnaise
150 ml/¼ pint plain yoghurt
1 tablespoon lemon juice
½ teaspoon horseradish
salt and freshly ground black pepper, to taste

1   Mix all the ingredients together well.

Beanpole Salad

Serves 2

1 small ripe avocado, peeled, stoned and diced
juice and zest of 1 lemon
175 g/6 oz beansprouts
120 g/4 oz sweetcorn – from a tin, or frozen, then
  cooked
50 g/2 oz button mushrooms, sliced
1 × 200-g/7-oz tin tuna (in brine or water)

1   Place the avocado in a large bowl with the lemon juice
     and zest.
2   Add the remaining ingredients and fold together, trying
     to forget everything your origami teacher ever taught
     you.

Sandwich Bar

Before you go rushing off to fill a whole French stick as your
sandwich, it's a couple of slices of bread only. If you have the
sandwiches open, though, you can pile them up higher!

RED LIGHT – steak, mayonnaise, cheese slabs, chip butties,
crisps, lamb and pork chops, sausages. Need we say more?
AMBER LIGHT – a piece of lean, thinly sliced roast beef,
peanut butter, lean ham, slimly sliced cheese. Get the
picture?
GREEN LIGHT – heaps of salad things, hummus, low-fat

cream cheeses, cottage cheese, tuna, salmon, thinly sliced chicken and turkey, a small tin of low-sugar baked beans. That'll do nicely.

Gotta Be Cruel to Be Kind

Spot the puddings! You're right, there aren't any. When you're dieting, the only way not to look like a pudding is not to eat them. While you're being strict, it's best to stick to fruit, the occasional low-fat yoghurt or a couple of dried figs or apricots to satisfy a sweet tooth. Having said that, a sweet treat every now and then is OK. Don't feel guilty if you give in.

CHAPTER SIX

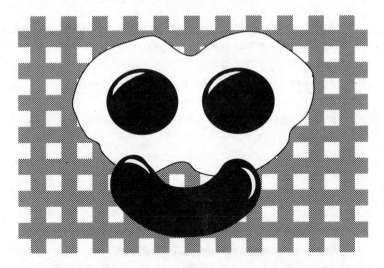

No More Yawning in the Morning

Here's a quick quiz to find out what sort of shape you're in.

Do any of the following statements apply to you?

1   *I have a whole wardrobe of clothes a size too small for me which I keep promising myself I will slim into.*
    Yes   No
2   *I sound like a steam engine after I've walked up a flight of stairs.*
    Yes   No
3   *The last time I went to an aerobics class I was the*

flabby one at the back in a baggy tracksuit who kept getting the moves wrong.

Yes   No

4   I would rather miss the bus than run for it.

Yes   No

5   People keep asking me if I'm preparing for hibernation.

Yes   No

6   I need a zimmer frame whenever I go out on the dance floor.

Yes   No

7   The last time I took any form of exercise was playing for the school tiddlywinks team.

Yes   No

8   I lose 8 pints of sweat just vacuuming the carpet.

Yes   No

OK, *now* go back and answer truthfully.

If you answered 'yes' six times or more, you're the original couch potato. If you had two to five 'yes' answers, you're probably some sort of relative of Wayne or Waynetta Slob. One 'yes' or all 'nos' is just the job, but are you movin' and a-shakin' as much as you could be?

GET IN SHAPE WITH SONGS BY:
THIN Lizzy, SLIM Whitman, LITTLE Richard, LITTLE Eva, The SMALL Faces, MINNIE Ripperton, Adam ANT, the Electric LIGHT Orchestra, Stiff LITTLE Fingers, BONEY M, Mother Love BONE, LITTLE Feat.

A Mover and a Shaker

Others call it exercise. We call it movin' and a-shakin', because on the *Big Breakfast* Fitness Plan, working out is FUN – almost as much fun as trying to remember the ABBA members' Christian names.

Here are a few reasons why YOU won't be able to resist getting physical every morning:

🖒 it's more fun-packed than a sausage

🖒 it helps you lose weight and stay trim

🖒 it boosts your spirits and helps you deal with stress a lot better

🖒 it makes your skin glow

🖒 it builds up your self-esteem as you start to like what you see in the mirror

🖒 you'll have more zest for life

🖒 you'll be able to keep up with the pace of the *Big Breakfast* antics

🖒 you'll have a leaner, firmer body with no wobbly bits (i.e. not like Sean the cameraman's)

🖒 your heart will get broken less easily as it will be so much stronger

🖒 you'll be the first to reach the bargains at sale time

Convinced about the benefits? Now here's how to get started.

EXERCISE MYTH

No pain, no gain. This is a big fat lie. If it hurts, stop at once!

Nice and Easy Does It

The first steps you take to get fit should be nice and easy, just like an old Frank Sinatra song. It's far better to start up really slowly, say with ten minutes of movin' and a-shakin' a couple of times a week. Gradually build up so that after two months or so, you're up to thirty minutes a day, three times a week (or more if you get hooked). And if you want a good excuse to slot your fitness session into your day, why not work out as you watch *The Big Breakfast*? Besides, getting moving first thing in the morning guarantees you'll be full of beans all day!

Opportunity Knocks

There are so many different ways of getting moving. Some don't even seem like exercise:

☞ *Let the dog take the lead* . . . Yes, walking the dog is as good for you as it is for your favourite pooch — providing you let him pull you along and put a bit of energy into it.

☞ *Get in the swim* . . . If you have kids, chances are they'll love swimming too, so it's a way of getting the whole family fit. To make swimming reach the parts that haven't been reached for a long time, try to vary your strokes so you use different muscles, and also swim as fast as you can.

☞ *On yer bike!* . . . Try riding a bike to work, to the shops or even just for fun at the weekend. It's absolutely fab for flabby thighs and big bottoms.

☞ *Cor, what a luverly pair of rollers* . . . Not Carmens, not Royces, but skates.

☞ *In a league of your own* . . . Team sports – from football and rugby to softball and netball – are ideal for improving fitness levels. Er, that's playing, not watching. Being part of a team means you're less likely to drop out of training sessions or matches because you can't let the side down.

☞ *Dancing in the street* . . . in a club, in the front room or in your bedroom. Wherever you do it, really go for it. Get steamy and sweaty with a salsa. Lambada your way to lithe and lean. Develop rock-solid muscles with rock 'n' roll. How many other diet books encourage you to party?

☞ *Top of the class* . . . There are also bound to be plenty of fitness classes on offer at your local sports centre or gym – a good way to meet new people as well as shape up.

And now for something completely different.

SUPER-HINT

When you're waiting for a bus or train, sneak in a Standing Bum Clench. Stand straight, feet slightly apart, and hold in your stomach muscles. Then clench your bottom as hard as you can. Hold for a few seconds, then relax and repeat ten to fifteen times. Try to look casual while doing this. Don't grit your teeth or hold your breath so you go red in the face.

SUPER-HINTS (your indispensable guide to getting moving and keeping it up)

🖐 *It's a goal! Your motivation could be wanting to lose a stone, run a mile or do up the zip of your size twelve trousers. Make a list of your goals, both short- and long-term, then give yourself a reward when you score them (no, not Maltesers). And make sure everyone knows how well you're doing – there's no substitute for a pat on the back. But remember, giving away too many penalties means going into extra time to burn up that blubber.*

🖐 *Don't be a half-baked being. Take a tip from Heinz, who swear by 57 varieties to keep in good shape. Madonna also follows the variety-is-the-spice-of-life principle – one day she weight trains, the next she swims, then she cycles and so on. Varying the activities means you won't get bored doing the same old thing and you'll get more all-round fitness benefits.*

🖐 *All you have to do is believe (and all your dreams will come true) ... Try to think yourself fit. This means doing things to improve and enjoy your performance like imagining you're winning a race while you jog round the park.*

🖐 *Do it for fun as well as for your figure. Life is too short to stuff too many mushrooms. Get on with physical activities you enjoy and don't force yourself to take part in something you hate or you'll never stick at it.*

Kidding Around

When you're looking for exercise inspiration, think back to your childhood and the fun you used to have messing around in the playground or street. It might surprise you, but getting fit can be as easy as ABC.

SPACED OUT

Remember Spacehoppers, those big orange bouncy things? Well, you can still buy them in toy shops and they're totally brilliant to work out with. You probably won't want to bounce into work on one (unless you're called Skippy), but try Spacehopping around the garden or up the street. It tones up your legs, works wonders for your inner thigh muscles and does quite a bit for your bum too. At first aim to bounce for at least ten minutes, working your way up to twenty minutes.

HU-LA-LA

Yes, a hula-hoop can be part of your fun fitness routine too. Keep it spinning round and round by wiggling your hips and waist. It'll work your stomach muscles and waist and the front of your thighs and your bottom, if you bend your legs and do it with a bit of control. Try it for a few minutes, till you get the knack, then do it for as long as you're still having fun. Not recommended if you've got a bad back, though.

TRIM ON THE TRAMPOLINE

Mini trampolines are available in sports shops and department stores all over the country and cost around £40. Just set one up in your front room and dance to music. Do the locomotion, twist, pogo or whatever makes you feel good. Or you could bounce on it while you watch *The Big Breakfast*. Vary your steps by jogging on the spot, jumping with both feet together and high-kicking with alternate legs. Draw the curtains while you do it so your neighbours think you've got a really exciting secret!

SUPER-HINT

Don't forget to keep breathing steadily while you work out. It might sound silly, but lots of people hold their breath, then end up panting and feeling exhausted.

YOU CAN SKIP THIS BIT

Fooled you, this one's about getting sweaty with a skipping rope. Boxers do it a lot, as it's an essential part of their fitness routine. It gives the heart and lungs a great workout and shapes up your legs, bum and shoulders. If skipping on your own, a good rope helps, so choose one with weighted handles. Once you've got the hang of it again, make the moves more interesting by landing on alternate feet or jumping with both feet together and then turning the rope backwards. Keep your arms close to your sides and turn the rope with wrist action, not your whole arm.

You could also rope some friends in and 'play' skipping with more people, just like in the school playground – a really different kind of mass workout from an aerobics class. Skipping isn't recommended, however, if you have back, knee or Achilles tendon problems.

THE TRUE MEANING OF CLEANING

So maybe it's a chore, but doing housework is also a way to fight the flab if you put enough elbow grease into it. Discover the virtues of vacuuming as you shimmy around unpiling the pounds. Feel that body move! Dust dynamically and give your arms a good stretch and tone. Washing up can be a wonderful workout too. Really!

To burn up 100 calories, you need to:
IRON for 52 minutes
SCRUB THE FLOOR for 16 minutes
SWEEP THE FLOOR for 30 minutes
VACUUM for 38 minutes
POLISH FURNITURE for 52 minutes

ONE OR TWO GREAT STEPS FOR MANKIND

Getting fit can be as easy as simply putting one foot in front of the other. Just be natural and don't overstretch. To be more energetic, make marching movements with your arms – swing those limbs. Get fitter by going faster and further each time you do a walk.

ONE STEP BEYOND

If you want to take up jogging, don't force yourself to jog the whole distance before you're fit enough (and end up with egg on your face because you can't do it). Start with a few minutes or paces of walking, then jog, then walk again. Soon you'll be able to jog all the way.

RUNNING ORDERS

☞ *Don't put your foot in it – get a decent pair of trainers for essential support and cushioning.*

☞ *Be safe. Never run in deserted areas, even in day-light, and don't wear a personal stereo – you need to be able to hear what's going on around you. A friend on the way keeps muggers at bay, so get someone to run with you if you can. You can encourage each other to keep moving too!*

☞ *For jogger's nipple and other jogging nasties, slap some Vaseline on anywhere where your skin is rub-bing or chafing.*

☞ *If you're bigger than Pavarotti, have medical prob-lems, say with your heart, or are very unfit, check with your GP before taking up running or indeed any exercise programme.*

☞ *Running water – have a few sips before and after running to avoid getting knackered and really thirsty.*

BORN TO RUN

Here's how to get the fun runs . . . Take things slowly. Pretend you're Anneka Rice and set yourself a challenge, such as running for ten minutes three times a week. By simply adding a minute or two on each session per week, you should get to the stage by week eight, nine or ten where you're running three times a week for twenty minutes. Interestingly, if you didn't stop the watch at ten weeks, you'd get to the point where you'd be so busy running you wouldn't have time to go to work or do the washing up. Before you go off running, don't forget to do some stretching (*see* page 109).

SPOTTY BOTTY?

For the smoothest baby-soft skin, you should slough off the dead skin cells. It's not as painful as it sounds. There are special products on the market called scrubs or exfoliators, which you just apply to the skin, massage around with a bit of water, then wash away. You can do it with a handful of salt too, slightly dampened before you start massaging. Don't scrub so hard that you make your bum go bright red, though!

THE **BIG** BREAKFAST DIET

Ten-Minutes-to-Breakfast Tone-Up

Try this simple set of exercises to strengthen and tone your
muscles. Don't forget to warm up first (see page 109). As you
get fitter, repeat all the exercises two or three times.

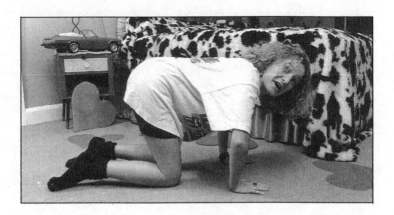

THE WIMP'S PRESS-UP

Get on the floor, on your hands and knees just like Lisa, who
works in the *Big Breakfast* phone room. Your knees should
be directly below your hips, your hands in line with your
shoulders. Keeping your back straight and your bottom out,
bend your arms at the elbow and dip your head and upper
body towards the floor. Repeat ten times. If you really want
to show off, or you're ready to progress, you can do the full
press-up with your legs straight out behind you.

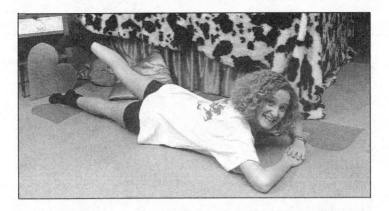

THE 'IT'S CHEAPER THAN LIPOSUCTION' BUM LIFT

Lie on the floor, on your stomach, with your forehead on your hands (not raised like Lisa's). With your toes pointing down to the floor, slowly raise your left leg up as far as you can, but without lifting your hip from the floor. Lower and repeat ten times before changing to your right leg.

THE SADDLE-BAG SHIFTERS

Part One: this works your outer thigh. Lie down on the floor on your left side with your head on your left arm, which should be stretched out above your head. Bend your right arm in front of your body with your palm on the floor to provide balance. Point your toes and lift your right leg about ten inches, then lower it again. Do this ten times. Your knee should be facing forwards as you lift, i.e. don't roll it so it

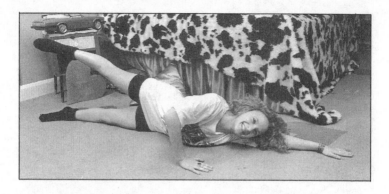

faces the ceiling. Roll over on to your right side and repeat the movements with your left leg.

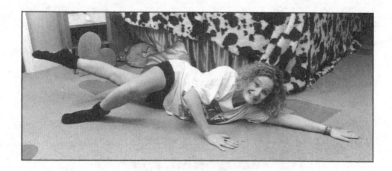

Part Two: this works your inner thigh. Lie on your left side with your head resting on your left arm (head *down*, Lisa!) which should be stretched out in line with your body. Put your right hand in front of you for support. Bend your right leg in front of you, but don't let the knee touch the floor. Now lift your bottom leg (the left one) up and down ten times. Turn over and repeat with your right leg.

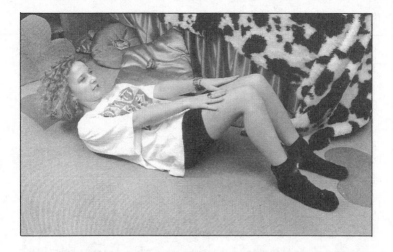

THE SPARE-TYRE PUNCTURE

Lie on the floor, flat on your back, with your knees bent and slightly apart. Press your lower back into the floor. Place your hands on the top of your thighs and gently lift your shoulders from the floor so your hands move towards your knees. Keep your head relaxed, your chin off your chest and use your stomach muscles to give the movement. Lower and repeat ten times.

CHAPTER SEVEN

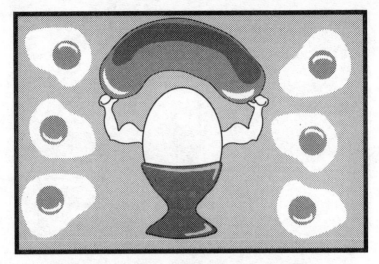

Eggstra Eggsercise

Inspired? On the way to becoming a cereal exerciser? Here are three fast, fun routines you can do at home at any time of the day to hone that physique into unbelievable shape. *The Big Breakfast* crew had a go (recognize them in the pictures?) — if *they* can, *anyone* can! Don't forget to warm up first with the Flex and Stretch moves (see opposite).

The first two routines are toning exercises. They shape you, but they don't work your heart and lungs and burn up a lot of energy, like running, swimming and Spacehopping do. Ideally, for your figure and your health you should combine both types of activity.

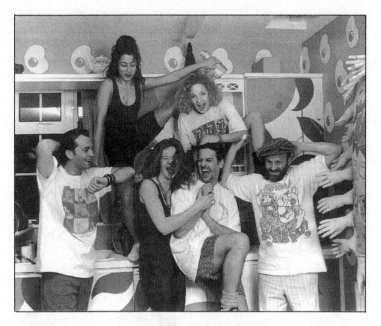

FLEX AND STRETCH

Before any kind of exercise, it's important to do a few flexibility moves and stretches. You should definitely do them before attempting the Tums, Bums and Thighs routine (page 125), the Awesome Beach Body Workout (page 125) and the Boxercise (page 139). The moves warm up your muscles, reduce risk of injury and protect against muscle soreness later. They also impress anyone who happens to be watching. The stretch session suggested below will take between five and ten minutes. It's actually quite a good routine to do as soon as you get out of bed, even if you're not going to do any real exercise.

1   Walk around the room or on the spot for four to five minutes without feeling remotely silly or once thinking

'Why am I doing this?' Increase your speed and incorporate arm movements until you feel warmer.

2 Do the following stretches, two to three times each and hold them for at least eight seconds each.

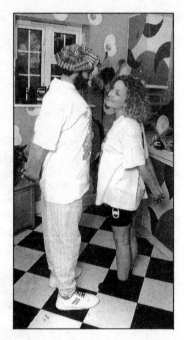

☞ Stand straight, feet slightly apart, knees relaxed (i.e. not locked tight). Roll your shoulders, circling them up and back. Then circle up and forwards. Turn your head to the right, hold, back to the centre, then left, hold. It's important to keep your eyes off the television at this point as the sight of the Family of the Week having a huge fried breakfast could break your delicate concentration.

☞ Bend your left arm behind your head so your hand touches your right shoulder. Reach up with your right hand and gently pull on your left elbow. Hold, then repeat swapping arms.

☞ Clasp your hands behind your back and push your shoulder blades together like Val and Lisa are doing (above). Now pull your arms up behind you. Hold. Reverse this move by clasping your hands in front of you at shoulder level, palms facing out. Push forward, rounding your back, dropping your head slightly. Hold (opposite).

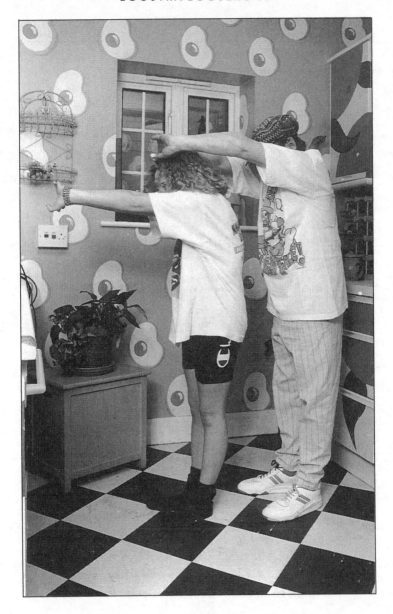

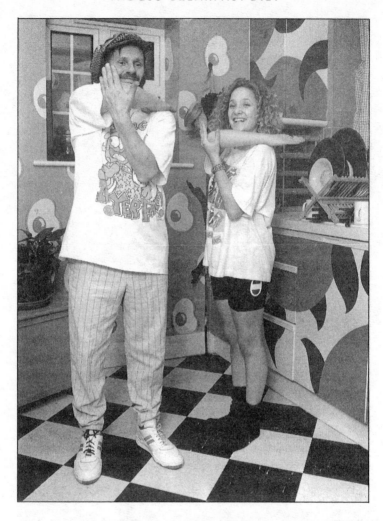

☞ Bend your right arm in front of you so your hand rests on your left shoulder. Using your left hand push gently on your right elbow so it moves towards your left shoulder. Hold and repeat on the other side.

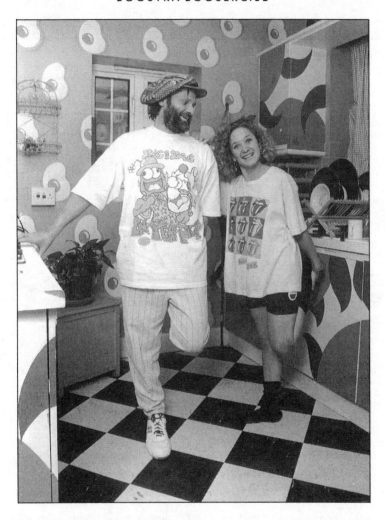

☞ Stand straight and bend your left leg behind you, holding the ankle with your left hand. Pull your foot towards
your bottom and hold. Repeat with the right leg.

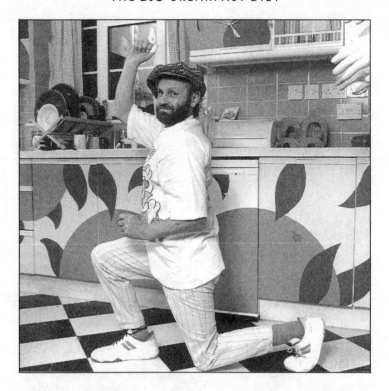

☞ From the standing position, take a big step forward (the trailing foot should remain on the ground). Allow the knee of the trailing leg to rest on the ground. Your front leg should be bent, so your knee is in line over your foot. Hold, then return to the start position and change legs.

☞ Standing straight again, step backwards and bend your back leg. Extend the other leg in front of you with the heel on the floor, toes pointing up. Your body will naturally lean slightly forwards. Now flex and point your foot several times, holding each movement.

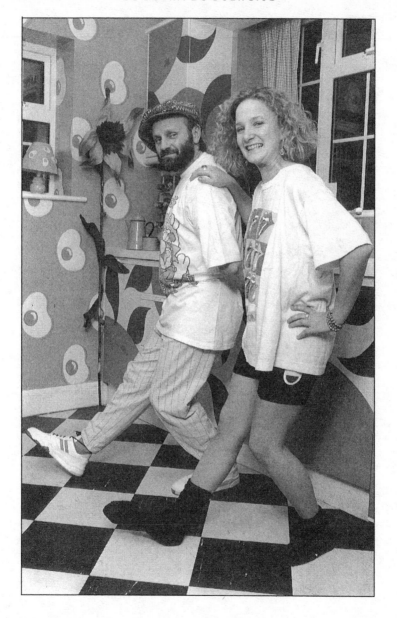

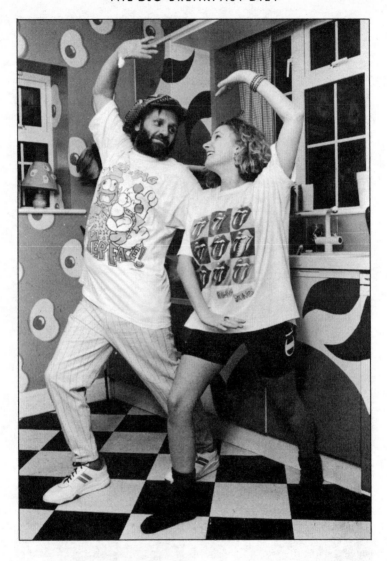

☞ Back to the upright standing position. This time take a
step forward and bend your front knee so it is directly in

line over your foot. Keep the back leg straight and your heel flat on the floor (like Val's). Shift your weight on to the back heel and push slightly forward with the front knee. Hold. Change legs and repeat.

The Awesome Beach Body Workout

Picture this ... warm blue sea, sand that's almost too hot to walk on, a gentle breeze, the smell of sun-tan lotion ... and you, looking an awesome beach babe (or dude). OK, so maybe it wasn't like that last year, but this year things are different. You've been following the *Big Breakfast* healthy diet, you've started to lose a couple of pounds and you're feeling full of energy and enthusiasm. Right, you reply in a breezy voice which smacks healthily of garlic and the juice of raw vegetables. Now here's the shape-up plan that will put the others in the shade, while you are the most gorgeous thing on the beach.

HOW TO DO THE WORKOUT

As you'll see from the photographs starring Ed, the *Big Breakfast* runner, the exercises in this section use weights to add resistance while you're working your muscles. Run through the exercises a couple of times without weights to get familiar with the routine. You'll still feel those muscles working and it will have an effect. After a few trial runs, incorporate the weights. You could use tins of food or other household items that are easy to grip – for instance, the unopened tubs of chocolate spread you have cleverly failed to eat. Doing the exercises with weights of 1–2 pounds is marginally better than doing them with no weights at all.

To really maximize the benefits you need to work out with the right weight for you. As a rule of thumb, if you can't do eight repetitions of an exercise then the weight is too heavy for you. If you can do more than fifteen easily, it's probably not heavy enough. Two to three pounds may be right for a woman to start off with and five pounds for men, but this will of course vary with individuals. By the way, women shouldn't worry about building bulky muscles. Unless you're also taking male hormones, steroids or training for hours on end with really heavy weights, there's no way you will end up looking like a body-builder!

Try to do ten to fifteen repetitions of each exercise. Then move quickly on to the next one. Aim to complete the whole circuit once, or twice if you are using very light weights. Do also try to copy the positions accurately, both for safety and effectiveness.

As this is a toning routine, for all-round fitness and for boosting your metabolism, you should also try to do some aerobic exercise. That means walking, running, playing a sport or doing an aerobics class two or three times a week.

THE WORKOUT

1 The Suitcase Lift

(works the front of the thighs and buttocks)

(a) Stand with your feet just further than hip-width apart, your toes turned out, arms at your sides holding the weights.

(b) Now bend your legs, keeping your knees aligned over your feet. Tightening your thighs and buttocks, straighten back up to the start position in (a).

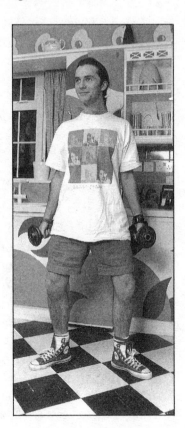

2 Lunge to the Sun
(works the front and back of the thighs and buttocks)

(a) Stand facing a low bench or step, feet hip-width apart, toes pointing forwards. Try not to lock your knees. Hold the weights in your hands by the sides of your body.

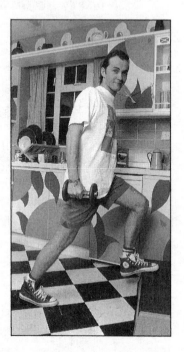

(b) Lunge forward with your left leg so your left foot is on the step. Your left knee should be directly in line over your left foot. The angle of your thigh to calf should be 90 degrees. Now push off the step with your left foot, squeezing your bum and thigh muscles while straightening your left leg out. Return to the start position and change legs to repeat the movement on the other side. Now, if nothing appears to have snapped or handed in its resignation, move on to the next exercise.

3 At Their Peak
(works the muscles around the chest)

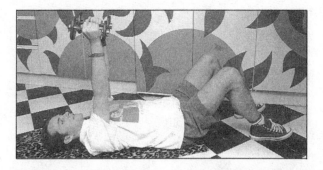

(a)   Lie on your back on the floor, with your knees bent, feet flat on the floor, hip-width apart. Press your lower back into the floor. Lift your arms up straight in front of you, holding the weights in your hands. Your palms should be facing each other.

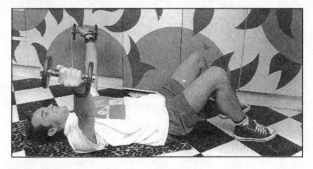

(b)   Slowly open your arms out to the side, keeping your elbows slightly bent. Then, slowly and with control, lift your arms back up to the start position (a).

4 The Water-Skier's Shoulder Raise
(works the muscles around your shoulders)

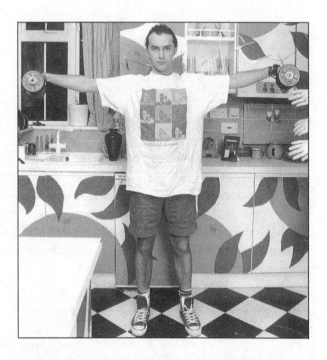

(a) Stand with your feet slightly apart and your knees relaxed (i.e. not locked). Hold the weights at your sides, but don't lock your elbows. Your palms should be facing your thighs.

(b) Lift your arms up out to the side until they're in line with your shoulders. Your elbows should still be slightly bent and your palms will now be facing down towards the floor. Slowly lower your arms back down.

5 Tenerife Triceps

(works the muscles at the back of the upper arms)

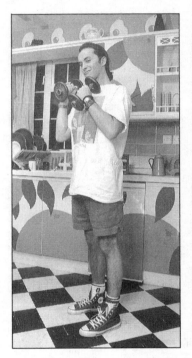 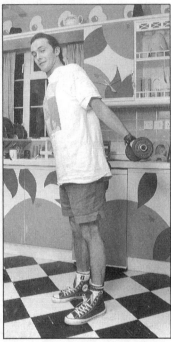

(a) Stand with your feet a little apart, with your elbows bent, as shown, holding the weights next to your chest. Your palms should be facing each other. (Ed really fancies himself as a macho man here.)

(b) Now straighten your arms behind you by pushing the weights back. While doing the movement, make sure your elbows are kept close to the sides of your body. Go back to the start position.

6 Scare the Wimps off the Sun-Loungers
(works the muscles at the front of the upper arms)

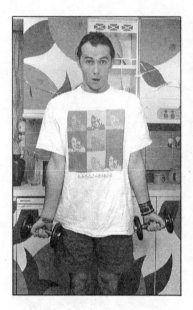 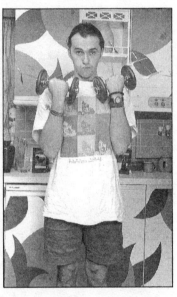

(a)   Standing as shown or seated with a straight back, hold the weights in front of you, holding your elbows close to your sides. Your palms should be facing forwards.

(b)   Bend both arms so the weights move up towards your shoulders. Then lower them again slowly. You could also alternate your arms so that one hand at a time moves towards your shoulder. Ensure that whichever way you do it your elbows stay close to your sides throughout.

Thanks to Peter Bissell, Fitness Manager at Henlow Grange Health Farm, for these awesome exercises.

Well done! You're alive. Now you can put your weights down and do the stomach exercises in the Tums, Bums and Thighs workout.

AWESOME BEACH BODY

How to look like an extra from *Baywatch* – don't call, it's just for fun . . .

1   Do our Awesome Beach Body Workout.
2   Apply fake tan. All over.
3   Run down a beach in slow-motion.
4   Wear a red swimsuit/red trunks wherever possible.
5   Paint your car yellow and write *Baywatch* on the side.
6   Take swimming lessons.
7   Don't take any acting lessons.
8   Be born with big teeth.

How to look even more AWESOME . . . Learn to surf, windsurf, water-ski or play beach volleyball.

Tums, Bums and Thighs

A characteristic of the British woman is a tendency towards the pear shape, i.e. heavier down below than on top. It's actually quite normal and natural to store fat around the tummy and bottom area. And, despite popular diet-speak, a tum that's flatter than a week-old can of Coke is not part of a woman's physiological make-up. However, having a couple of spare tyres can and should be avoided! You can do exercises to tone up these wobble-prone areas and, of course, if you eat sensibly you won't pile on the pounds there either.

HOW TO DO THE WORKOUT

The following routine should be done as a complete circuit. Do it once all the way through, aiming for ten to fifteen repetitions of each exercise. Once you can do that easily, progress to doing the whole routine twice.

Men can do these exercises too, to avoid a 'beer belly' (or, if it's too late for the word 'avoid' to have any meaning, let's say 'to enter into negotiations with your beer belly') and squidgy bum and thighs.

Remember that these are toning and shaping exercises, which for maximum results and all-round fitness should be combined with regular aerobic exercise.

TUMS

1 Tilt that Tum

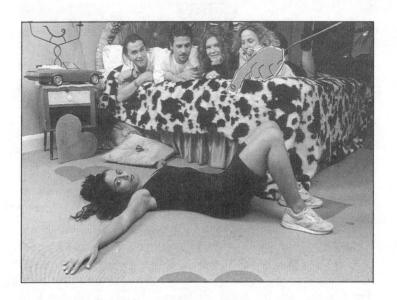

Lie on your back like the *Big Breakfast* runner Jasmine with your knees bent and your feet flat on the floor. Put your arms out to the sides so they're in line with your shoulders. Breathe in, then breathe out while pulling in your tummy muscles and pushing your lower back into the floor. Breathe in and relax.

2 The Curler

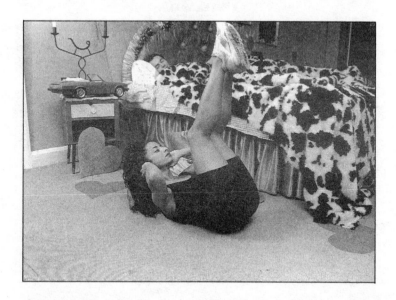

For this one, you're in the same position as for Tilt that Tum except this time bend your arms behind your head as shown. Carefully curl up so your head and shoulders rise off the floor. As you lift, make sure your lower back is firmly pressed into the floor and that your tummy muscles are held in tightly. Breathe out as you lift up, and in as you lower slowly back down. To progress you can lift up higher so that your upper back comes off the floor too.

3 One Tum or Two?

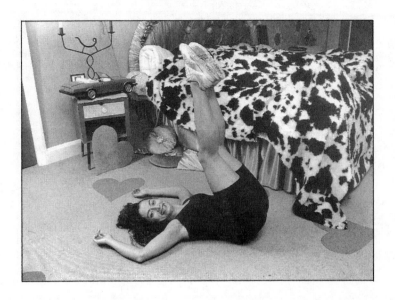

Lie on your back with your legs up so your knees are over your tummy. You can put your arms at your sides or behind your head. Breathe out and pull in your tummy muscles while trying to lift your bottom an inch or two off the floor (your lower back, however, should stay firmly on the floor). Breathe in as you lower back down.

4 Defining the Lines

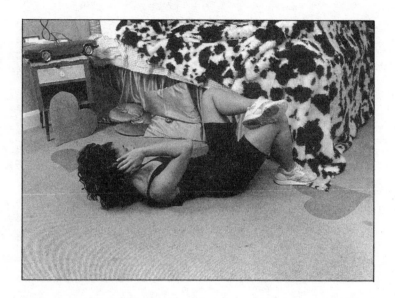

Lie on your back with your right knee bent so your foot is close to your bottom. Bend your left leg so your left ankle rests over your right thigh. With your right hand bent behind your head, breathe out and slowly lift up, reaching towards your left knee with your right elbow and shoulder. Lower back to the start position while breathing in. After doing the repetitions, swap sides so you reach with your left elbow to your right knee.

5 When It Comes to the Crunch

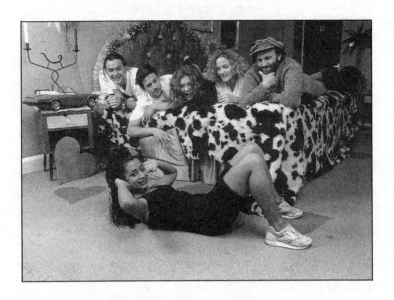

For the crunch, you're in the same position as for One Tum or Two? except your hands must be behind your head, fingers touching loosely. Breathe out and lift your head and shoulders up off the floor while holding your tummy muscles in tightly. At the same time pull your knees towards your chest. Breathe in as you lower back down.

BUMS

6 Bye-Bye Big Bum

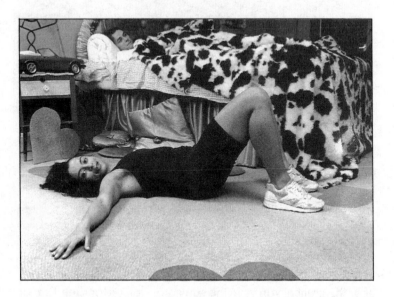

Get into the pelvic tilt position as in Tilt that Tum, but have your arms closer to your sides. Now squeeze your bum tight and lift it a few inches off the floor. Hold for a few seconds, then relax back down.

7 Hands, Knees and Bums-a-Daisy

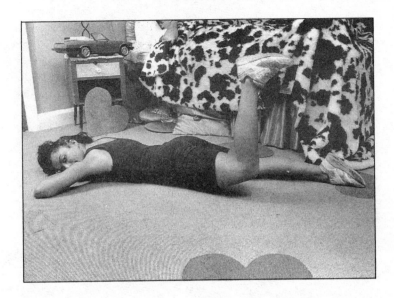

Lie on your stomach with your head resting on your arms in front of you. Keep your right leg straight and bend your left knee so your leg is at a 90-degree angle. Keeping your hips on the floor, tighten your bum and lift your left knee a couple of inches up off the floor. Slowly lower and repeat.

8 The Bottom Line

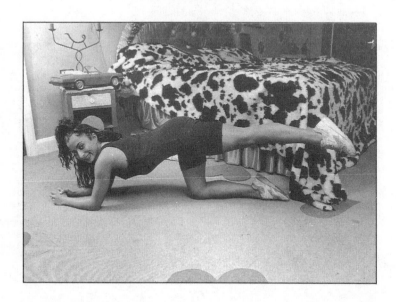

Position yourself as shown, leaning on your elbows and forearms and with your left leg stretched out behind you, toes on the floor. Now lift your left leg up (toes pointing down towards the floor) so it's in line with your hips. Lower it to the floor, but don't let your toes quite make contact with the floor before you lift again. Repeat with right leg.

OUTER HIP, THIGHS AND BUM

9 Thigh-High

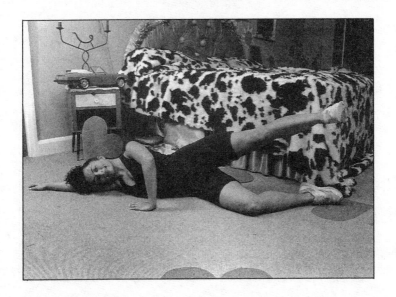

Lie on your right side with your right leg slightly bent and forward. Stretch your left leg out, with the foot flexed so your toes are pointing forwards, i.e. facing the same direction as your body. Now lift up your left leg in a small movement, then lower. Change sides and repeat.

10 The Thigh's the Limit

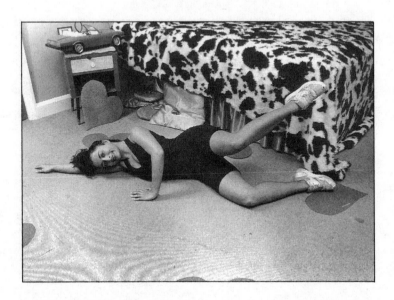

Lie on your right side with both knees bent and forward so they're in line with your hips or lower. Lift your left leg up 6–12 inches, lower and repeat. Change position after doing your repetitions so that you work the right leg too.

INNER THIGHS

11 The Legover

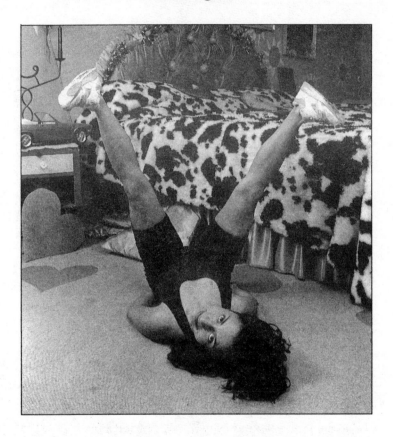

Lie on your back with your hands under your bum, palms on the floor. Put your legs up in the air so that they're directly over your tummy. Feet together. Now slowly move them as far apart as feels comfortable. Then draw them back together.

137

FRONT OF THIGH

12 Gladiator Thighs

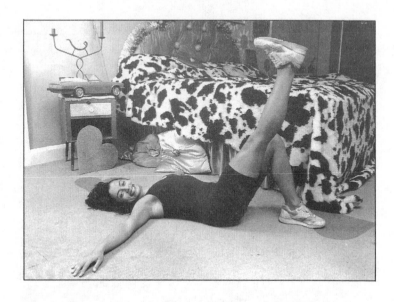

Lie on your back as for the pelvic tilt position in Tilt that Tum. Straighten your right leg along the floor, toes pointing towards the ceiling. Now lift it an inch or two off the floor. Then, with your lower back pressed firmly into the floor, lift the straight leg up 2 or 3 feet (so it makes a 45–60 degree angle with the floor). Lower the leg so it nearly touches the floor, then raise it again. Repeat with the left leg.

Bums, Tums and Thighs firmed up with exercises by Peter Bissell, Fitness Manager at Henlow Grange Health Farm.

Boxercise

The trendiest way to work out since 'the Step', Boxercise combines boxers' training moves with a circuit of exercises. It's fast, challenging, totally different and lots of fun (Rob the cameraman and Ronnie the AFM certainly thought so). Best of all is to do it in a class situation, where you have all the equipment and a professional instructor. Classes are starting to spring up all over the country, so make a mental note to look out for one in your area.

The following routine has been put together by Paul Connolly, an ex-Amateur Boxing Association champion and gym instructor. It's a taster of the sort of thing you'd find in one of his Boxerobics™ classes, run in London and Essex. This workout tones you up and also gives you a cardiovascular session, so it's unbeatable for getting you fighting fit!

HOW TO DO THE WORKOUT

For this one you do need a bit of 'equipment':
- ☞ a skipping rope
- ☞ a rope or string, about 6 feet/2 metres long
- ☞ stairs or a step
- ☞ a sturdy chair
- ☞ a mirror, preferably full-length
- ☞ a football
- ☞ dumbbells or strap-on weights, or, in an emergency, tins of food
- ☞ a sparring partner

The exercises or 'rounds' should each be done for ten to thirty seconds before you move on swiftly to the next one. It will take a while to master the moves, but don't let that put you off. And don't forget to warm up first.

THE WORKOUT

Round One – Triceps Dips

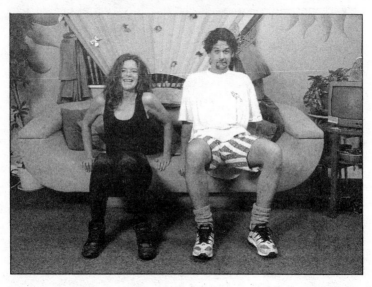

Position yourself with your back towards a chair, the palms of each hand on the edge of the seat. Put your feet flat on the floor, knees bent at a 90-degree angle. Straighten your arms, but don't lock your elbows. Make sure there's a little space between you and the chair. Bend your arms and lower your body so your elbows are level with your shoulders. Then push back up to the start position.

Round Two – Standing Hooks to Mirror

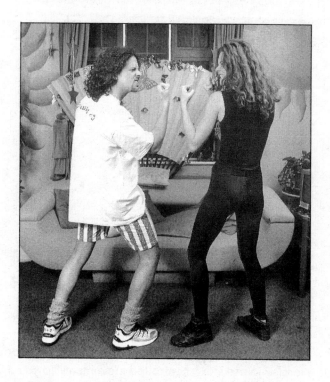

For this you need a full-length mirror to stand in front of. Stand with your feet just further than hip-width apart, form fists and bend your elbows with your arms in front of you (i.e. just a like a boxer). Use a hooking motion and swing your fists, one at a time, at an imaginary target in front of you (or you can do it with a partner, like Rob and Ronnie). As you find momentum, your hips will move from side to side in a steady rhythm. The power for this move comes from your upper, outer back, under the arms and down your sides.

Round Three – Up and Overs

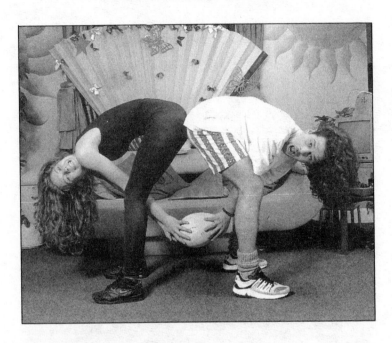

You need a partner for this one. Take care too when doing this exercise to use slow, controlled movements so you don't hurt your back. Stand back to back with your partner, knees slightly bent and legs wide enough apart to allow a football to pass through (or in this case a papier mâché ostrich egg – and why not?). The person who starts with the ball should bend carefully from the waist to pass the ball through their legs and into the other person's hands. You should then both raise yourselves upright and stretch your arms up fully to pass the ball back over your heads. Repeat for half the time, then swap the direction of the ball-passing.

Round Four – Skipping

If it works for Mickey Rourke, it could work for you. This helps your cardiovascular system and improves coordination, footwork and balance. Skip, holding the rope quite close to your sides. Wrist movement rather than whole-arm movement should swing the rope. With your feet together, make small side to side jumps, but try to keep your upper body in the same position as you skip.

Round Five – Seated Ball Twists

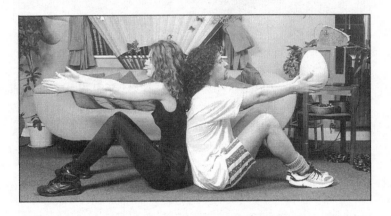

This is not as painful as it sounds! Sit back to back on the floor with your partner, with your lower backs pushed together, knees bent and feet flat on the floor. One of you should start with the ball, arms straight out in front of you with the ball at chest height. Keeping the ball at the same height, slowly turn your upper body until your partner (who should copy your move as if in a mirror) gets the ball. Your

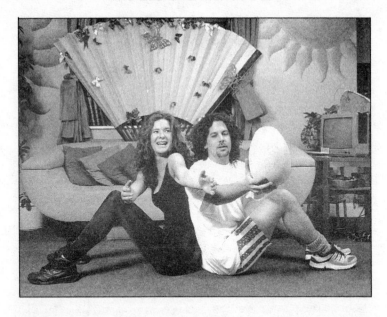

partner should then slowly turn to the other side (as should you) and pass the ball back to you again. Continue passing the ball in this direction for half the time, then reverse the direction.

Round Six – Rope Ducks with Upper Cuts

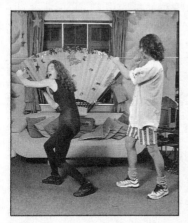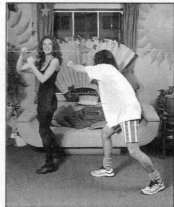

Fasten the rope at shoulder-height and stand at one end of it. Make a fist with the hand furthest away from the rope, then move in sideways, ducking under the rope. After ducking, straighten up and throw an uppercut punch. Work along the rope, ducking and always punching with the hand furthest from the rope.

Round Seven – Football Drop

One person should lie flat on the floor with their knees bent and hands at the sides of their stomach. The other person stands above you, their legs either side of your hips. The person standing holds the ball, which they will aim and drop (not throw) at the stomach of the person on the floor. Incidentally, the higher the drop, the harder 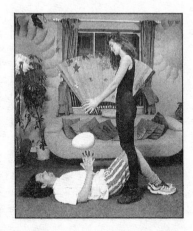 the exercise. As the ball falls, the person on the floor should flex their abdominals and catch it, absorbing as little or as much of the ball's weight as they feel comfortable with. Once the ball is caught it should be thrown back up to the person who's standing.

Round Eight – Step-Ups

Stand in front of a stair or, if you have one, a step. Step up on to the stair with your right foot and follow it with your left so both feet are on it. Step back down, first with your right foot, then with your left. Alternate the leading leg and repeat the movement rhythmically.

Round Nine – Snatch and Press

Hold hand weights/dumbbells/food tins in both hands and from a standing position bend your knees to a 90-degree angle, keeping your back straight, bum out and head up. In one movement bring the weights to shoulder-height, straightening your body. Now push the weights above your head, straightening your arms. Lower them back to the shoulder position, then bend your legs and bring them back down, but don't let them touch the floor.

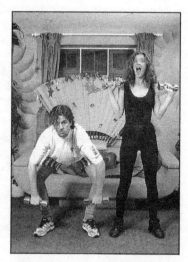

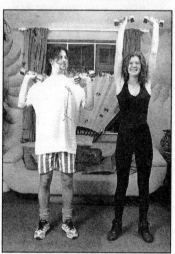

Round Ten – Football Sit-Ups (or the Terry Venables)

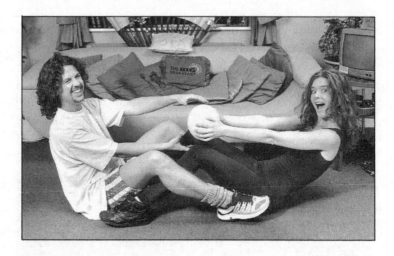

Sit facing your partner with your legs interlocked and one of you holding the football to your chest. Now pass it to your partner. Both of you should now lower yourselves to the floor, slowly, vertebra by vertebra. When your shoulder blades touch the floor start to come up again, using your stomach muscles as opposed to the strength of your legs. The ball should now be passed back again.

Round Eleven – Shadow-Boxing to Mirror

Stand in front of the mirror. The instructions here are for a right-handed person (an orthodox boxer), so reverse them if you're left-handed (a south paw). Stand left side on to the mirror and make fists with your hands, bringing them to face-height. Keep your left arm in line with your body and bring your head down, tucking your chin into your left shoulder. Bring your right arm up so your hand covers the right side of your face. Now lean forward on the balls of your feet, which should be roughly hip-width apart. Your heels are off the floor to allow a pivoting movement. Lead with a left jab and follow with a right cross.

Round Twelve – Rapids with Hand Weights

Hold the weights in each hand and jog on the spot. Slowly increase your speed and the height of your legs so they're almost at chest-height. After ten to thirty seconds, jog down slowly, lowering your knees. Put your weights down and walk on the spot for another few minutes.

To finish, do the stretches described at the beginning of this chapter (page 109).

CHAPTER EIGHT

A Week in The Life of a Big Breakfast Dieter

It could look something like this:

	Breakfast	**Lunch**	**Dinner**
Sunday	The Lovers' Breakfast, with an extra piece of fresh fruit	The Sunday Roast	Large mixed salad, with 2 slices wholemeal bread with a non-meat spread
Monday	A breakfast cereal with skimmed milk and 1 piece fresh fruit	Blow-Your-Socks-Off Chilli, with rice	It-Won't-Show-on-the-Scales Minestrone and Slimline Smoked Mackerel Salad
Tuesday	Our Daily Bread	Grilled white fish, with potatoes and veg	Very Orange Soup and Totally Tropical Salad

A WEEK IN THE LIFE OF...

	Breakfast	*Lunch*	*Dinner*
Wednesday	A Caribbean Breakfast	Baked potato with any topping plus extra vegetables if you like	Large mixed salad, with 2 open pile-'em-high sandwiches
Thursday	A breakfast cereal with skimmed milk plus 1 piece fresh fruit	Chicken Chegwin, with rice or potatoes and vegetables	Down Mexico Way salad, with 2 slices of bread
Friday	The Go-Faster Breakfast	Dish the Fish, with rice or potatoes and vegetables	Goodness Greekcious, with pitta bread and dip
Saturday	The Cholesterol Get Losterol Breakfast plus 1 piece fresh fruit	Lean-i Fettuccini	Skinny Soup and Tabbouleh to Go

And another week could look something like this:

	Breakfast	*Lunch*	*Dinner*
Sunday	Kedgeree-Do	To Be or Nut To Be, with piles of vegetables	Large mixed salad, plus 2 slices wholemeal bread
Monday	The 'Behind Enemy Lines' Breakfast	Baked potato with any topping	Magical Mushroom Soup and Tabbouleh to Go
Tuesday	A breakfast cereal with skimmed milk and 1 piece of fresh fruit	Grilled chicken breast with potatoes and vegetables	Beanpole Salad, with 2 slices of bread
Wednesday	The White-On Breakfast	Pasta with any topping	Very Orange Soup, and 2 open pile-'em-high sandwiches
Thursday	The Big Chill Breakfast	Lock-Keeper's Mackerel, with potatoes or rice and vegetables	Goodness Greekcious, with 2 slices of bread

A WEEK IN THE LIFE OF...

	Breakfast	*Lunch*	*Dinner*
Friday	Our Daily Bread	Fill It with Millet	Skinny Soup and Pounds-Away Pasta
Saturday	Mega-Mix Muesli	Bikini-Friendly Blinis	Down Mexico Way salad, plus 2 slices of bread

And of course there's more to it than food. Here are some nice-and-easy ideas on how to get moving this week.

Sunday   Get your partner to MASSAGE you before, during or after your Lovers' Breakfast

Go for a SWIM, a long country WALK or JOG down to your local sports centre or gym to find out what's on offer there. Don't stop at the pub for a quick pint on the way back.

Monday   WALK to work, the station or the shops. And back again.

Tuesday   BOUNCE on a mini trampoline for ten minutes while watching *The Big Breakfast*, or do the HU-LA-LA with a hula-hoop or try the TEN-MINUTES-TO-BREAKFAST TONE-UP.

Aim to WALK at a fast pace for ten to twenty minutes too – whether it's during your lunch break or some other part of the day.

Wednesday   Give yourself a salty body scrub before your bath or shower (see page 103) so your skin feels as smooth as silk.

Go for a brisk ten- to twenty-minute WALK, JOG or RUN around the park.

Thursday   Ready to give the TUMS, BUMS AND THIGHS routine a whirl? Go on, you can do it.

Friday   Dance, dance, dance.

Saturday   Facemask time. Slap on a ready-made one or try the DIY recipe on page 39.

Repeat the TEN-MINUTES-TO-BREAKFAST TONE-UP. Also go for a long WALK, BIKE RIDE or SWIM, attend an AEROBICS class or try an exercise video at home.